Get Fit!

How To Gain The Freshman 15 Of Muscle

Arielle Tolbert

Ordering Information

Special discounts are available on quantity purchases by corporations, associations, and others. For details, contact the publisher at the address above.

Printed in the United States of America

First Printing 2017

978-0-692-85651-2

www.ArielleTolbert.com

ABOUT THE AUTHOR

Arielle Tolbert's a Computer Engineering major at Michigan State University whose modeling and acting career began at 16.

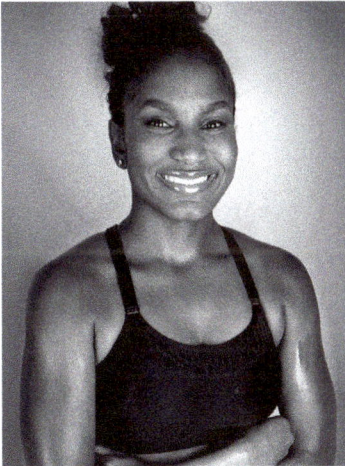

Health and fitness is a true passion for Arielle. She's considered the YMCA her "second home" since her early teens and enjoys eating healthy, working out, and inspiring others to do the same.

As she says, "I hope to help people fall in love with a healthy lifestyle."

That's why she became a personal trainer, group fitness leader, and wrote this book.

Arielle is also the creator and co-host of the weekly "Fire & Ice Conversations" webcast which tackles tough topics and increases awareness of important, often-overlooked, community issues.

SPECIAL THANKS

I would like to give special thanks to Uncle Brian, Michelle, and all of my family and friends for their love, support, and encouragement. I could not have written this book without you all!

HOW TO USE THIS BOOK

The purpose of this book is to help college students get and stay fit while enjoying their college experience.

It's a guide to the foundation needed to start a healthy lifestyle during college and maintain that lifestyle when you graduate and move onto your next endeavors.

CONTENTS

AUTHOR'S NOTE

As a college student, it is easy to fall into a pattern of poor lifestyle habits. The constant stress of balancing classes with a social life can take a toll on eating, sleeping, and fitness habits—or lack thereof.

That is why I wrote this book: as a guide to prevent students from falling into this easy yet unhealthy lifestyle and reverse the habits of those who may already have been trapped.

The title of my book says "How to Gain the Freshman 15...of Muscle"—but this book is about more than building muscle.

It's a guide to eating healthy, losing, maintaining, and gaining healthy weight, turning body fat into muscle, and working out, all while maintaining a balance of classes and social life.

This book is not just a bunch of words—it is my own testimony, researched and tested in my own life.

I implemented the very things I've written here into my life: eating healthy, working out, and balancing classes and my social life. I even indulged in some unhealthy foods, but I got right back on track and managed to decrease my body fat percentage a total of 6%. This book is flexible enough to cater to your personal needs and goals. All you have to do is be willing to make lifestyle changes and build new habits.

The key to this change is to gradually remove unhealthy foods from your diet in order to see more definition in your muscles and reduce those layers of fat. Then, once you feel that you have reached your level of desirable muscle definition, you can gradually indulge in unhealthy foods—in moderation and on occasion.

This book helps you answer the ultimate question:

> Do I want to gain the "freshman 15" of muscle...or the "freshman 15" of fat?

UNDERSTANDING YOUR BODY

It is important to remember that your body is not about the number on the scale; rather it is about the amount of fat on your body.

Muscle weighs more than fat. That is why when you weigh yourself after working out and eating healthy, you may notice an increase in the scale. When this happens, remember that you are not gaining fat, but muscle. Your body is essentially about how you look and feel when your body is bare and you are absolutely naked.

As you embark on this journey towards a healthy lifestyle, take note of the way you look and feel currently—whether you take a picture or document your body fat percentage. Use this moment in the beginning of your journey to track your progress and measure how close you are meeting your goal.

Body fat is classified using the following body

fat percentage chart:

Classification	Women	Men
Essential Fat	10-13%	2-5%
Lean	14-20%	6-13%
Average	21-24%	14-17%
Acceptable	25-31	18-25%
Obese	32%+	25%+

You can calculate your current body fat percentage using a fat loss monitor, body fat calipers, or a tape measure and record it below.

Current Body Fat %: _____

As you read the following chapters, understand that everyone has a different body type. What works for someone else may not work for you.

PART 1: HOW TO ACHIEVE PROPER NUTRITION

College has easy access to almost any food you want—at any time. This makes it easy to make unhealthy food choices. Eating healthy is all about portion sizes, nutrients, calories, and timing.

Tackling Portions

According to the Merriam-Webster dictionary, a portion is enough food, especially of one kind—like protein, or carbohydrates—to serve one person at one meal.

These simple guides can help you estimate suitable portion sizes using your finger, thumb and hand:

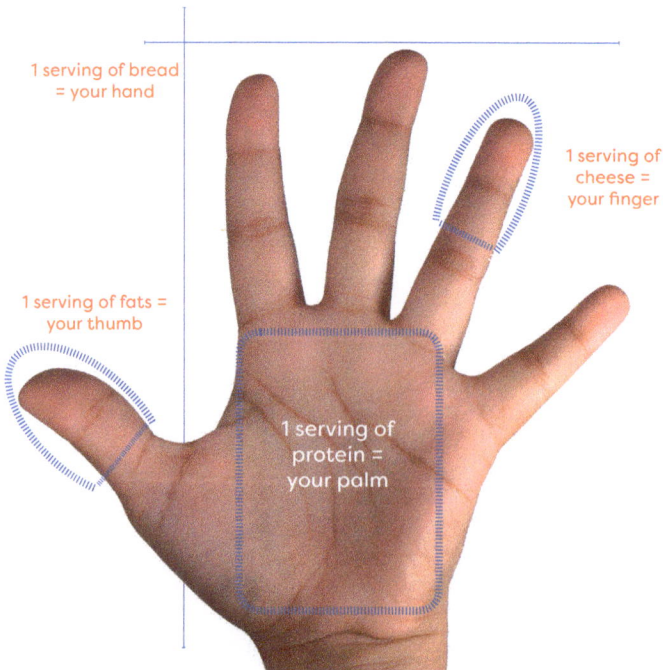

1 serving of bread = your hand

1 serving of cheese = your finger

1 serving of fats = your thumb

1 serving of protein = your palm

You can use your fist to estimate portions for foods like these:

1 serving of vegetables, fruits, milk,
yogurt, cooked noodles, grains, or cereal
= your fist

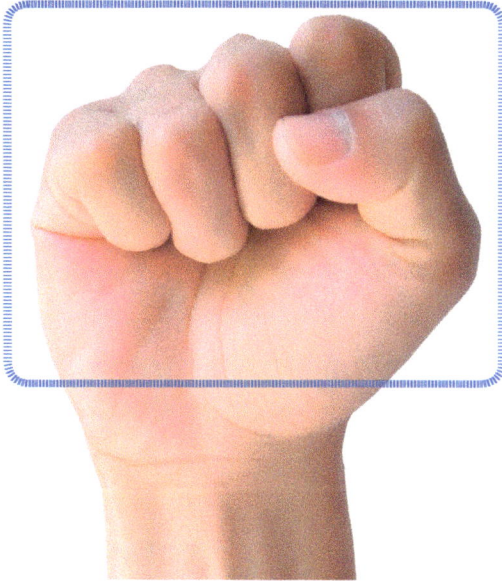

What Should I Eat?

Eating the right portion size—just enough, not too much, not too little—is important for your health.

Too much of a certain amount of food can be bad for your body. You are eating to fuel your body. Eating the proper type and amount of foods will give your body the nutrients it needs.

To maintain a healthy diet, you need the proper combination of proteins, carbohydrates, fats, vitamins & minerals, and water, as the plate below displays:[1]

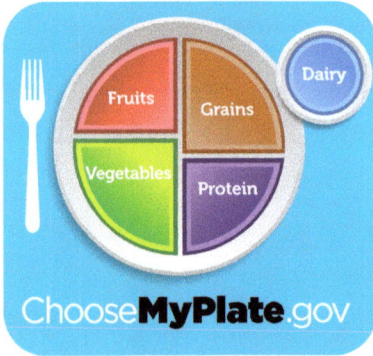

Proteins	12%
Dairy	15%
Fruits & Veggies	33%
Grains	33%
Fats	7%

The following are a few examples of what to look for, from each type of food, in the cafeteria and in your normal diet.

Proteins

Proteins and water make up muscle, which is why protein is a key component in your diet.

The main function of protein is to support the growth and repair of body tissues, which is why protein needs vary per person.

The following chart gives some examples of key proteins from both animal and vegan sources that you can look for.

1 *MyPlate Graphic Resources: Choose MyPlate.* (2016, Dec. 16). USDA Center for Nutrition Policy and Promotion.

ANIMAL	VEGAN
Lean Meat	Seeds
Seafood	Peas
Poultry	Nuts
Eggs	Peanut butter
Low-fat dairy	Dried beans
	Lentils

Carbohydrates

Carbohydrates (carbs) are essential for the body because they provide the body with the energy it needs to function. However, beware of bad carbs that don't offer any nutrients at all. More than half of your plate should be fruits, vegetables, and grains like these:

GOOD CARBS	BAD CARBS
Fruits	Refined sugars
Vegetables	Artificial sugars
Whole grains	Molasses
Dried beans	Alcohol
Oats	High fructose corn syrup
Peas	Corn syrup
Lentils	
Raw honey*	

* Raw honey is a healthier option than sugar, but too much honey leads to the negative effects of bad carbs.

Fats

Contrary to popular belief, fats are needed to help your body function in many ways.

Fats provide backup energy when carbohydrates are not available and absorb essential vitamins for the body that help preserve healthy skin and hair.

Stored fat also surrounds and protects vital organs and insulates body temperature.

Although "good" fats are essential, only a small amount of such fat is needed to maintain good health.

Here are a few examples of good and bad fats and where to find them.

GOOD FATS	BAD FATS
Monounsaturated fats	**Saturated fats**
Avocados, almonds, cashews, hazelnuts, sesame seeds, canola oil, olive oil, peanut oil	Eggs, high-fat dairy products, beef, pork, chicken with skin, coconut oil
Polyunsaturated fats	**Trans fats**
Fish: catfish, salmon, trout, tuna	Baked goods, butter, fried foods, packaged foods, microwave popcorn, some margarines
Nuts: walnuts, pistachios	
Vegetable oils	

Vitamins & Minerals

Vitamins and minerals like vitamins A, B, C,

D, E, and K, keep your body strong, healthy, and in tip-top shape.[2] By eating a balanced healthy diet, your body will be receiving all the vitamins and minerals it needs to be fit.

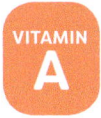

VITAMIN A Vitamin A supports the maintenance of teeth, skin, bones, vision, and muscle membranes. It's found in:

LIVER, MILK, CHEESE, CARROTS, SWEET POTATOES, EGGS, PUMPKIN, KALE, PEACHES, CANTALOUPE, APRICOTS, PAPAYA, MANGOS

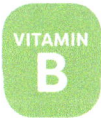

VITAMIN B Vitamin B supports the metabolism, proteins, hair, skin, nails, red blood cells, energy conversion and the nerve system. Look for it in:

WHOLE GRAINS, LIVER, PORK, NUTS, SEEDS, SOYBEANS, EGGS, MILK, CHEESE, YOGURT, DRIED BEANS, MUSHROOMS, PEANUT BUTTER, MEAT, FISH, POULTRY, ENRICHED GRAINS, BANANAS, POTATOES, OATMEAL, CHICK PEAS, LENTILS, PISTACHIO, SUNFLOWER SEEDS, WATERMELON, CAULIFLOWER, CARROTS

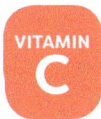

VITAMIN C Vitamin C supports teeth, gums, body tissue, hair, nails, the breakdown of fatty and amino acids, and wound healing, and can be found in:

---

2 "Vitamins: MedlinePlus Medical Encyclopedia." (2015, Feb. 2.) Retrieved Aug. 2, 2016 from https://medlineplus.gov/ency/article/002399.htm

KIWI, STRAWBERRIES, MANGOES, PAPAYA, BROCCOLI, BRUSSELS SPROUTS, TOMATOES, BROCCOLI, SPINACH, CITRUS FRUITS AND JUICES

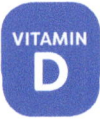

VITAMIN D

Vitamin D supports teeth and bones. You'll find it in:

EGGS, SALMON, TUNA, SARDINES, MILK, SOY MILK

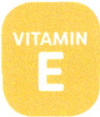

VITAMIN E

Vitamin E supports red blood cells and is an antioxidant for the body. It's found in:

AVOCADOS, VEGETABLE OILS, NUTS, LEAFY GREEN VEGETABLES, WHOLE GRAINS, WHEAT GERM, PEANUT BUTTER

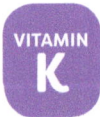

VITAMIN K

Vitamin K supports blood clotting and can be found in:

BROCCOLI, KALE, SOYBEANS, COLLARDS, TURNIP GREENS, SPINACH, BEET GREENS, FISH

Water

Water is vital for healthy eating, because water makes up more than half of the human body.

On average, 8 glasses of water per day is needed to maintain a healthy diet. More accurately, your amount of water intake is based on your weight and level of exercise.

To determine your recommended baseline daily water intake, divide your body weight in half and that answer will be your specific water intake in ounces.[3]

_____ lbs ÷ 2 = _____ oz. water/day
BODY WEIGHT

Then, factor in the amount of exercise you engage in per day. This can be done by multiplying the amount of minutes you exercise by 12, dividing that result by 30, and adding your final answer to your baseline daily water requirement:

$$\frac{\text{\# exercise minutes} \times 12}{30} + \text{Baseline Daily Water Intake} = \underline{\quad} \text{ oz. water/day}$$

Tackling Calories

A calorie is the measurement of energy. Since the amount of energy needed to function differs per each body, the average amount of calorie intake varies per person:[4]

---

3 Stone, J., PT, DPT. (2014, Jun. 19). *How to Calculate How Much Water You Should Drink.* Retrieved Feb. 28, 2017 from https://www.umsystem.edu/newscentral/totalrewards/2014/06/19/how-to-calculate-how-much-water-you-should-drink/
4 *Estimated Calorie Needs per Day.* USDA Center for Nutrition

Average Daily Calories For Women		
	Age 18	Ages 19-25
Less active	1,800	2,000
Moderately active	2,000	2,200
Active	2,400	2,400

Average Daily Calories For Men			
	Age 18	Ages 19-20	Ages 21-25
Less active	2,400	2,600	2,400
Moderately active	2,800	2,800	2,800
Active	3,200	3,000	3,000

These averages may not take into account extremely short or extremely tall body types because muscle mass is an additional factor, due to the fact that muscles constantly burn calories.

The key to **losing** weight is to decrease the amount of calories obtained from bad carbs, fat, and empty calories by 500 and to make sure that the amount of calories burned is greater than the amount of calories consumed.

The key to **maintaining** weight is to balance the amount of calories burned to the amount

Policy and Promotion.

of calories consumed.

The key to **gaining** weight is to increase the amount of calories obtained from foods high in nutrients, like proteins, good carbs, and healthy fats and to add more resistance training to your workout.

Generally, 3,500 calories equals about one pound of fat, which breaks down into 500 calories per day. Each of the following food examples averages about 500 calories. Just cutting back on one of these foods each day adds up to 3,500 calories each week.

500-Calorie Examples

1 regular plain bagel + cream cheese

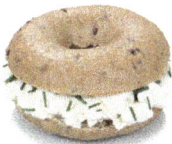

2 regular doughnuts

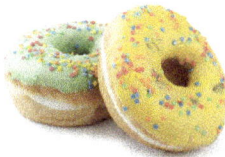

1 peppermint hot chocolate mocha

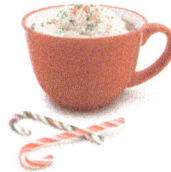

4 slices of bacon

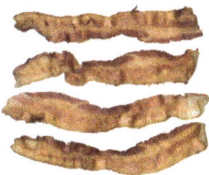

2 regular candy bars

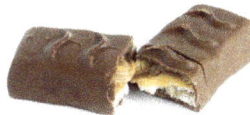

Managing Calorie Intake

Eating smaller portions and staying away from empty calories—like alcohol, candy, soda, and chips—can help you manage your calorie intake.

However, if you want to specifically log the amount of calories from each food you eat or manage the nutrients you have received, you can use tools like "My Fitness Tracker," "Super Tracker," or "Ipiit, The Food Ambassador."

Tackling Labels

Many people consume enough, if not more, of their daily calories, without consuming their necessary daily nutrients.

One way to reduce this is to use food labels to understand the amount of servings and the type of ingredients and nutrients a certain food provides.

It is also important to remember to stay away from artificial ingredients like additives and preservations.

How do you identify these artificial ingredients?

Simple.

If you cannot pronounce the ingredient or do not know what it is, you do not want it in your body.

The following example of the nutrition label for ramen noodles shows you how to read food labels.

Once you understand the information food labels contain, you can use it to make better food choices.

Sample Label: Ramen Noodles

❶ SERVING SIZE

This is the first thing you need to look at when looking at a label. The "serving size" tells you the amount in a serving, and the "servings per container" tells you how many of those "serving sizes" are in that single package. Here you can see that 1 serving is equal to half a dry block of Ramen Noodles or 1.5 ounces.

② CALORIES

You then look at the amount of calories and calories from fat that are in each serving. It is important to remember that servings with:

- ⊙ 40 calories or fewer are low in calories

- ⊙ Around 100 calories are reasonable in calories

- ⊙ 400 calories or more are high in calories

Since there are 60 calories from fat out of the total 190 calories in the serving, the amount of calories is reasonable. However, 32% of those calories are from fat.

③ UNHEALTHY NUTRIENTS

After looking at the serving size and calories, you then need to look at the amount of unhealthy nutrients that is in each serving.

Remember that these nutrients are not completely bad for you. However, they need to be very limited in your diet in order to maintain proper health. As you see in the label, 7 grams of total fat and 910 milligrams of sodium is present in each serving.

④ HEALTHY NUTRIENTS

This section shows you the amount of healthy nutrients in each serving. Unlike the unhealthy nutrients that you want to limit, these nutrients should be abundant in your diet to improve your health. Therefore, you can see that 2 grams of fiber, 5 grams of protein, and 10 percent of your daily iron consumption goal is present in one serving.

5 % DAILY VALUE

This information tells you how much each nutrient uses from your caloric intake per day.

The percentage of daily value is calculated out of 100% of the assumed calorie diet given on the label. Therefore, based on the percentage of daily value given, you can determine if a nutrient is high or low in a serving.

- ⊙ A daily value of 5% or less is low

- ⊙ A daily value of 20% or more is high.

According to the label, 11% of your total 100% limit of total fat per day is used, 38% of your 100% of total sodium allowance is used, and only 10% of your total iron goal of 100% is used per serving.

6 RECOMMENDED DAILY CONSUMPTION

You can also look at the footnote at the bottom of the label to tell you how much of each nutrient you should include or restrict in your daily diet.

Now, let's look at ramen noodles overall.

The good news is that it's cheap, and fairly

low in calories.

It also provides a fair amount of iron. On the other hand, it doesn't have that much protein or fiber, so by itself it isn't a balanced meal.

However, if you are unable to make a healthier food choice, then you can incorporate other foods from the underrepresented food groups—like beans for protein or vegetables for carbs—in order to add more balance to your meal.

Tackling a Fast Metabolism

The key to a fast metabolism is timing.

Knowing when exactly to eat and what to eat are fundamental for establishing a faster metabolism.

What is good timing?

Contrary to popular belief, a healthy diet consists of 4-6 small meals a day, each meal spaced out in increments of 3-4 hours throughout the day.

Eating such meals frequently allows your body to process food and burn fat faster.

It is crucial when establishing a fast metabolism to constantly feed the body in small frequent meals vs. large sporadic meals.

Large sporadic meals and extreme dieting have a negative affect on the metabolism because it causes the metabolism to slow down, instead of increase.

Inconsistent meals cause the body to store more fat because it does not know when its next meal and source of nutrients is coming.

Eating a healthy breakfast is also essential for creating a fast metabolism because it is necessary to break the fast the body entered when the body was asleep, and to avoid constant food cravings throughout the day.

Supplemental vitamins & minerals and green tea, which contain caffeine and catechins, have also been proven to aid in creating a faster metabolism by at least 4%.[5]

Tackling Snacking

When your classes are close and you don't have time to eat a full meal, you can find healthy snacks to eat that will give you enough fuel to last you until your next meal.

Here are some examples of healthy and unhealthy snacks.

---

5 Manfredi, T, PhD. *How to Get a Super Fast Metabolism.* Retrieved Feb. 28, 2017 from http://www.healthguidance.org

HEALTHY SNACKS

Water

100% cranberry juice

Protein shakes

Low-fat milk

Trail mix

Fruit cup

Applesauce

Pumpkin seeds

Celery & carrots

Greek yogurt

Skinny Pop & low-sodium popcorn

Protein bars

Mini/string Cheese

Almonds, cashews & pistachios

Low-sodium jerky

Dried fruit & raisins

Peanut butter

Whole wheat pretzels

Fresh fruit

Banana nut muffin

Whole grain crackers

Veggie chips

Fruit chips

Dark chocolate

Graham crackers

Oatmeal

UNHEALTHY SNACKS

Soda

Juice

Energy drinks

Sports drinks

Candy

Chips

Cookies

Cakes

High-sodium foods

High-fat foods

* Sports drinks are good to use when working out, but not as a common, everyday drink because of their high levels of sugar.

Tackling Fast Food

When you don't have time to cook your own meals, or you just aren't feeling like going to the cafeteria to eat, sometimes you're going to want to grab some fast food.

Fast food is not the best option for a healthy

diet. However, you can almost always find healthier choices if you keep a healthy plate in mind.

Follow these quick guidelines to make the most out of an unhealthy situation.

- ⊙ **Keep the amount of calories per meal under 500 calories**. To achieve your fitness goal you must follow the caloric guidelines given to you on page 21. You do not want to waste your daily calories and nutrition portions on one meal.

- ⊙ Look for the foods higher in protein and lower in fats and bad carbs.

- ⊙ Be aware of **sodium**. Many fast food places love to overload on sodium. Try to minimize the amount of sodium you consume in your meal.

The following charts provide nutrition information for some of the healthier options with fewer than 300 calories at these common fast food restaurants:

- ⊙ McDonald's
- ⊙ Subway
- ⊙ Wendy's
- ⊙ Burger King
- ⊙ Chipotle

- ⊙ Taco Bell
- ⊙ Panera
- ⊙ Pizza Hut
- ⊙ Chick-fil-A

McDonald's

	Calories	Protein (g)	Fat (g)
4-Pc Chicken Nuggets	180	10	11
Bacon Ranch Grilled Chicken Salad (no bacon)	230	34	7
Fruit 'N Yogurt Parfait	150	4	2
Egg White Delight Mc-Muffin	250	17	8
Apple Slices	15	0	0
3-Pc Mozzarella Sticks	190	8	10
Hamburger	250	13	8

Subway

	Calories	Protein (g)	Fat (g)
Turkey Breast Mini Sub	180	10	2
Veggie Delite® Mini Sub	150	6	1.5
Chicken Noodle Soup	110	8	3
Turkey Breast Salad	110	12	2
Baked Lay's® Orig. Chips	120	2	3.5

Wendy's

	Calories	Protein (g)	Fat (g)
Artisan Egg Sandwich (no bacon)	290	15	13
4-Pc Chicken Nuggets	180	10	13
Grilled Chicken Wrap	270	20	11
Jr. Hamburger	240	14	10
Apple Slices	35	0	0
Small Chilli	170	15	5
Plain Baked Potato	280	7	.5
1/2 Power Mediterranean Chicken Salad	240	20	9

Burger King

	Calories	Protein (g)	Fat (g)
Garden Side Salad (no dressing)	60	4	4
Quaker Oatmeal-Maple	170	4	3
Egg & Cheese Crois-san'wich	300	11	15
4-Pc Chicken Nuggets	170	8	11
Hamburger	220	11	8
Motts' Harvest Plus Applesauce	50	0	0

Chipotle

	Calories	Protein (g)	Fat (g)
Steak Burrito Bowl	150	21	6
Black Beans	120	7	1
Brown Rice	210	4	5.5
Lettuce	5	0	0
Fajita Veggies	20	1	.5
Green Tomatillo Salsa	15	0	0
Sofritas	145	8	10

Taco Bell

	Calories	Protein (g)	Fat (g)
Breakfast Soft Taco-Egg & Cheese	170	7	9
Fresco Chicken Soft Taco	140	10	3.5
Gordita Supreme-Chicken	260	16	9
Black Beans	80	4	2
Premium Latin Rice	100	2	2.5
Chicken Soft Taco	160	12	5

Panera

	Calories	Protein (g)	Fat (g)
Oatmeal w/ Almonds, Quinoa & Honey	300	8	6
1/2 Seasonal Greens Salad	90	2	6
1/2 Steak & Arugula on Sourdough	250	12	9
1/2 Roasted Turkey & Caramelized Kale Panini	300	14	11
Apple	80	0	0

Pizza Hut

1 medium slice	Calories	Protein (g)	Fat (g)
Ham & Pineapple (Pan)	230	10	9
Green Pepper, Red Onion, Diced Red Tomato (Fit 'n Delicious®)	150	6	4
Chicken, Red Onions, Green Pepper (Fit 'n Delicious®)	180	11	4.5
Supreme (Hand Tossed)	260	12	12
2-Pc Lemon Pepper Traditional Wings	150	8	10
2-Pc All American Traditional Wings	80	7	5

Chick-fil-A

	Calories	Protein (g)	Fat (g)
Sunflower Multigrain Bagel	220	6	3
Grilled Chicken Nuggets	140	25	3.5
Grilled Market Salad	200	25	6
Fruit Cup	45	0	0
Sm Kale Superfood Side	190	4	9

Tackling Nutrition During Breaks & Holidays

It's easy to establish an eating schedule at school and then get off track when going home for breaks due to homemade meals, large portions, and sometimes, lack of meals.

However, there are a few things you can do to in order to defeat those distractions.

Follow the advice given in this book to maintain a healthy diet

Include plenty of fruits, grains, vegetables, protein, dairy, and water. Constantly make an effort to ensure that as many of these food types as possible are included in your diet in moderation.

If your family is constantly into having homemade meals...

Get in the kitchen and encourage your family to eat healthier along with you. Recommend trying new recipes that are healthy yet still have that great "homemade" taste!

If your family always goes out to eat...

Always keep in mind what your "plate" is supposed to look like as shown in "What Should I Eat?" on page 15.

Many menus mention the "under 500 calories" entrees, "Weight Watchers" entrees, or make some type of note of the healthier options they offer at that restaurant.

If you cannot find those options, try to select an item on the menu that includes as much of your daily nutrients as possible without including a huge amount of sodium, bad carbs, and sugars.

If your family isn't really big on keeping the refrigerator full or making any meals at all...

Then take the initiative! Go out to the store yourself, or encourage your family to go to the store, and buy all the healthy food options that you want and feel that cater to you and your taste buds.

Remember, you must eat at least 4-6 meals a day in order to maintain a healthy diet.

This is a great time for you to discover and try new fruits, vegetables, healthy snacks, and recipes that you like and enjoy eating.

That way, you can know what works for you when it is time to go back to school!

PART 2: HOW TO FIND TIME TO WORKOUT

College life can be very demanding and time-consuming. This makes it easy to avoid working out. The key to finding time to workout is planning and prioritizing your schedule.

Planning & Prioritizing Your Schedule

In order to ensure that you will have time in your day to work out, you must pre-plan your schedule.

Planning your schedule allows you to not only know when certain events will occur during your day but also prioritize each event. Remember, at least 7-8 hours of sleep is very important in maintaining a healthy lifestyle.

Prioritize all the events in your schedule

Class

Work

Free time

Extracurricular activities

Homework & studying

Sleep

Workouts

Meals

Visualize your schedule

Use the following chart as an example of planning and prioritizing your schedule so that you will always have time to work out and sleep.

Execute your schedule.

Refer to page 58 to set up your own weekly schedule. You can also download PDF forms at ArielleTolbert.com.

Sample Schedule

	Sun	Mon	Tues	Wed	Thurs	Fri	Sat
8 AM							Free Time or Extra-curricular Activities
9 AM	Free Time or Extra-curricular Activities	Meal 1	Meal 1	Meal 1	Meal 1	Meal 1	
10 AM		Class	Class	Class	Class	Class	
11 AM							
Noon		Meal 2	Meal 2	Meal 2	Meal 2	Meal 2	
1 PM		Nap	Nap	Nap	Nap	Nap	
2 PM		Class	Class	Class	Class	Class	
3 PM							
4 PM		Meal 3	Meal 3	Meal 3	Meal 3	Meal 3	
5 PM		Workout	Workout	Workout	Workout	Homework	
6 PM		Homework	Meal 4	Homework	Workout		
7 PM			Homework	Meal 4	Meal 4	Meal 4	
8 PM		Meal 4		Extracur-ricular Activities	Homework		
9 PM							
10 PM							
11 PM		Sleep	Sleep	Sleep	Sleep	Sleep	

PART 3: TYPES OF WORKOUTS

Working out is more about your heart rate than the workout itself. In order to lose, maintain, or gain weight, one must not only workout but reach the target heart rate that caters to one's specific body type.

Determining Your Target Heart Rate

To determine your perfect workout, you must first determine your maximum heart rate. Input your age into the following equation to determine your maximum heart rate:[6]

220 – Your Age = Maximum Heart Rate

Based on your maximum heart rate, you can then determine your target heart rate zone using this equation:

Maximum Heart Rate x Target % =

Target Heart Rate

Use the appropriate Target % from this chart:

Zone	Target %
Warm-up & Cool-down	≤ 50%
Fat-Burning	50%-65%
Target Heart Rate	65%-85%
High Intensity	85%-100%

6 Karvonen, J. and Vuorimaa, T. (1988). Heart rate and exercise intensity during sports activities. Practical application. *Sports Medicine.* 5 (5): 303–11.

Understand Your Zones

Warm-up/ Cool-down Zone

In this zone, you increase your heart rate from its normal resting heart rate prior to your workout, and gradually decrease your heart rate to its resting heart rate after your workout.

Fat-Burning Zone

Here, the increase in your heart rate causes the fat in your body to be processed for energy use but does not create enough cardiovascular benefits for those who are looking to maximize calorie burning.

Target Heart Rate Zone

This zone is a moderate intensity activity level that is great for those who want to burn fat, lose weight, gain energy, and get fit.

High Intensity Zone

This zone is great for very athletic individuals. This zone has high intensity on the heart but does not burn a lot of fat, which is why it is great for training in short time intervals. For example, you can alternate between 60 seconds in the High Intensity zone, and 60 seconds in your Target Heart rate zone.

Determining Your Workout

A good workout can happen anywhere, not just the gym—on a field, in an open room, or even your dorm!

You must first create your workout! Training programs are also provided starting on page 48 if you need inspiration for your workout plan or just want something to get you started.

Create Your Perfect Workout

1. Answer these questions to get started:

- ⊙ How long do you want to work out?
  Ex: 1 hour

- ⊙ How often do you want to work out?
  Ex: 5 days a week, Monday through Friday

- ⊙ Which areas of the body do you want to target?
  Ex: Total body and core

- ⊙ Where do you want to workout?
  Ex: The gym

- ⊙ Do you want to use weights or dumbbells? If so, how much weight per exercise?
  Ex: Weights

2. Choose your exercises from the Exercise Directory that follows this section:

- ⊙ For a total body workout, choose

4-6 total body exercises and 2 core exercises

⊙ For an upper body workout, choose 4-6 upper body exercises and 2 core exercises

⊙ For a lower body workout, choose 4-6 lower body exercises and 2 core exercises

OR

⊙ Choose at least 3 upper body exercises, 3 lower body exercises, and 3 exercises that target your abs

3. Choose the number of reps and sets for each exercise:

⊙ 3 sets of 8-10 reps   ⊙ 4 sets of 15 reps

⊙ 3 sets of 15 reps   ⊙ 4 sets of 25 reps

⊙ 3 sets of 20 reps   ⊙ 5 sets of 8-10 reps

⊙ 4 sets of 8-10 reps   ⊙ 5 sets of 20 reps

Or create a workout combination of your own!

4. Write down your workout plan using the form on page 62 or download forms at ArielleTolbert.com.

Remember, no workout needs to be permanent to see results. Feel free to return to the Exercise Directory or add exercises of your own to switch up your workout any time!

Exercise Directory

Choose from these exercise examples to create the perfect workout that fits your schedule and location, and targets specific areas of the body.

You'll find photos of each exercise in the Exercise Gallery that starts on page 67.

CARDIO

Jog	Spinning Bike	Stair Climber
Jump Rope	Sprints	

TOTAL BODY

Blast-Off Push-Up	Jumping Mountain Climber	Side-to-Side Mountain Climber
Break Dancer	Karaoke	Skier Swing
Burpees	Low-Jumping Mountain Climber	Slam
Cross-Body Jumping Jack	Mountain Climbers	Speed Walkout
Diagonal Mountain Climber	Plank Jacks	Spider Mountain Climber
Face-Melter Step-Ups	Predator Jack	T-Rotation
Halo Slam	Push-Up Jack	Woodchops
High-Knee Run	Quad Push-Up	
Jumping Jacks	Seal Jack	

LOWER BODY

1 Leg Stand-Ups

Alternating Fast Feet

Alternating Lunges

Alternating Split Jump

Alternating Step-Up Jump

Ball Leg Curl

Box Squat Jump

Butt Kicks

Calf Raise

Deadlift

Donkey Kick

Double Fast Feet

Drop Step Back Squat

Dumbbell (DB) Split Squat

Fast Feet on Hands

Floor Touches

Front Squats

Front-to-Back Hop

High Kicks

In-And-Out Squat

Lateral 3-Step

Leg Extension

Leg Press

Leg Raises & Spreads

Long Jump & 3 Backward Hops

Low Box Lateral Runner

Low Box Runner

Low Rotational Chop

Lunge Runner

Lunges

Plyo Alternating

Plyo Single-Leg Hip Thrust

Pogo Jump

Power Skip

Prisoner Squat

Pulse Squats

Rolling Squat Jump

Running Lunge

Shuffle In Place

Side Lunges

Side-to-Side Hop

Single Leg Pogo Jump

Single-Leg Hip Thrust

Single-Leg Swing

Skater Jump

Sprinter Skip

Sprinter Step

Squat Hold

Squat Jacks

Squat w/ Leg Raise

Squat Walk

Squats

Sumo Squat

Super Skater Jump

Tuck Jump

UPPER BODY

Bench Press

Bent-Over Row

Chin-Up

Decline Bench Press

Dumbbell (DB) Curl

Dumbbell (DB) Curl & Press

Dumbbell (DB) Fly

Dumbbell (DB) Incline Press

Dumbbell (DB) Press

Dumbbell (DB) Side Raise

Front Raise

Hammer Curl

Incline Press

Inverted Row

Low Row

Machine Shoulder Press

Military Press

Overhead Tricep Extension

Plyo Clap Push-Up

Preacher Curl

Pull-Ups

Pull-Down

Punch

Push-Ups

Rear Delt Raise

Reverse Grip Pull Up

Seated DB Press

Seated Isolated Curl

Seated Tricep Dips

Shrugs

Tricep Dip

CORE

Ab Rollout

Bicycle Crunch

Bridges

Cable Crunches

Crab Touch

Decline Crunches

Flutter Kicks

Hanging Leg Raise

Oblique V-Ups

Plank Elbow Tap

Plank Hand Tap

Plank Hip Tap

Plank Knee Tap

Plank Row

Plank Shoulder Tap

Plank Speed Reach

Plank Toe Tap

Planks

Reverse Crunch

Rotational Chop

Russian Twist

Scissor Kicks

Side Plank

Side Plank Dips

Sit-Ups

Superman

V-Up

Weighted V-Up

Body Weight Program
About 30 minutes/day

Monday		Tuesday	
Floor touches	4x25	Floor touches	4x25
Burpees	4x25	Mountain climbers	4x30
Alternating lunges	4x30	Alternating lunges	4x25
Jumping jacks OR	3x50	Push-ups	4x16
Plank jacks	4x25	Jumping jacks	4x25

Wednesday		Thursday	
Floor touches	4x25	Floor touches	4x25
Burpees	4x15	Plank push-ups	4x30
Leg raises & spreads	4x15	1 leg stand-ups (each leg)	4x12
Jumping jacks OR	3x50	Mountain climbers	4x30
Plank jacks	4x25		

Friday		Daily Core Workouts	
Floor touches	4x25	Russian twist	3x50
Burpees	4x15	Plank	4x 1 -2 mins
Woodchops (each side)	4x15	Side plank dips	4x 1 -2 mins
Jumping jacks OR	4x30		
Mountain climbers	4x30		

Machine/Resistance Training Program 1
About 1 hour/day

Monday/Wednesday		Tuesday/Thursday	
Upper Body		**Upper Body**	
Bench press	3x10	DB incline press	3x10
Inverted row	3x10	Pull-down	3x10
DB incline press	3x12	Bent-over row	3x12
Chin up/pull-down	3x12	Push-up	3x12
DB side raise	3x15	DB curl & press	3x15
Push-up	3x15	Reverse grip pull-up	3x15
Lower Body		**Lower body**	
Alternating lunges	3x20	DB split squat	3x20
Box squat jump	3x15	Ball leg curl	3x15
Calf raise	3x10	Hanging leg raise	3x10
Core		**Core**	
Ab rollout	3x25	Plank	4x1 min
Russian twist	3x25	Side plank - each side	4x1 min

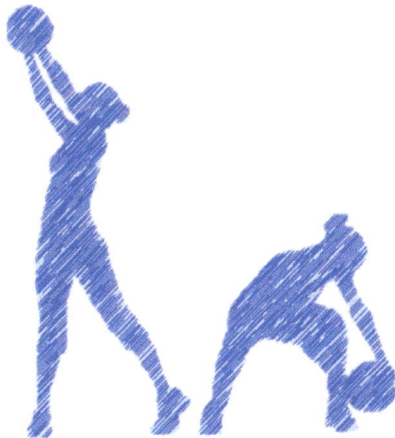

Machine/Resistance Training Program 2
About 1 hour/day

Monday		Tuesday	
Chest		**Legs**	
Bench press	4x10	Barbell lunge	4x10
Decline bench press	4x10	Single leg extensions	4x10
DB incline press	4x10	Ball leg curl (per leg)	4x10
Plyo clap push-up	4x10	Deadlift	4x10
		Calf raises	4x10
Shoulders		Barbell squat	4x10
Machine shoulder press	4x10	Sumo squat	4x10
Front raises	4x10	**Core**	
DB side raises	4x10	V-ups	4x10
Rear delt raise	4x10	Oblique v-ups	4x10

Wednesday		Thursday	
Arms		**Legs**	
DB curls	4x10	DB split squat	4x10
Isolated curls	4x10	Single-leg press	4x10
Tricep pull-down	4x10	Ball leg curl (per leg)	4x10
Tricep press	4x10	Deadlift	4x10
		Calf raises	4x10
Back		Leg press	4x10
Shrugs	4x10	Sumo squat	4x10
Pull-up	4x10		
Bent-over row	4x10	**Core**	
		Decline crunch	4x10
		Rotational chops (10/side)	4x10

30-Day Legs, Abs, Butt Challenge
About 30 minutes–1 hour/day

DAY 1	DAY 2	DAY 3	DAY 4	DAY 5
15 Squats 5 Bridges 10 Lunges 10 Ab rollouts	20 Squats 5 Bridges 10 Lunges 15 Ab rollouts	20 Squats 10 Bridges 15 Lunges 20 Ab rollouts	25 Squats 10 Bridges 15 Lunges REST	30 Squats 10 Bridges 20 Lunges 25 Ab rollouts
DAY 6	**DAY 7**	**DAY 8**	**DAY 9**	**DAY 10**
30 Squats 15 Bridges 20 Lunges 30 Ab rollouts	35 Squats 15 Bridges 20 Lunges 35 Ab rollouts	35 Squats 20 Bridges 25 Lunges 40 Ab rollouts	35 Squats 20 Bridges 25 Lunges REST	40 Squats 20 Bridges 30 Lunges 45 Ab rollouts
DAY 11	**DAY 12**	**DAY 13**	**DAY 14**	**DAY 15**
40 Squats 25 Bridges 30 Lunges 50 Ab rollouts	45 Squats 25 Bridges 30 Lunges 55 Ab rollouts	45 Squats 30 Bridges 35 Lunges 60 Ab rollouts	50 Squats 30 Bridges 35 Lunges REST	50 Squats 30 Bridges 40 Lunges 65 Ab rollouts
DAY 16	**DAY 17**	**DAY 18**	**DAY 19**	**DAY 20**
55 Squats 35 Bridges 40 Lunges 70 Ab rollouts	55 Squats 35 Bridges 40 Lunges 75 Ab rollouts	55 Squats 40 Bridges 45 Lunges 80 Ab rollouts	60 Squats 40 Bridges 45 Lunges REST	60 Squats 40 Bridges 50 Lunges 85 Ab rollouts
DAY 21	**DAY 22**	**DAY 23**	**DAY 24**	**DAY 25**
65 Squats 45 Bridges 50 Lunges 90 Ab rollouts	65 Squats 45 Bridges 50 Lunges 95 Ab rollouts	65 Squats 50 Bridges 55 Lunges 100 Ab rollouts	70 Squats 50 Bridges 55 Lunges REST	70 Squats 50 Bridges 60 Lunges 105 Ab rollouts
DAY 26	**DAY 27**	**DAY 28**	**DAY 29**	**DAY 30**
70 Squats 55 Bridges 50 Lunges 110 Ab rollouts	75 Squats 55 Bridges 65 Lunges 115 Ab rollouts	75 Squats 60 Bridges 65 Lunges 120 Ab rollouts	80 Squats 60 Bridges 70 Lunges REST	90 Squats 60 Bridges 70 Lunges 125 Ab rollouts

30-Day Full Body Program
About 1 hour/day

DAY 1	DAY 2	DAY 3
Push-ups 3x25 Pull-ups 3x15 Squats 3x12 Deadlift 3x12 DB press 3x12 Box squat jumps 3x35	Jumping jacks 3x50 DB side raise 3x20 Drop squat 3x30 Plyo clap push-up 3x12 Military press 3x12 DB curl 3x12/side	REST
DAY 4	**DAY 5**	**DAY 6**
Lunges 3x25 Squats 3x15 Lunge Runner 3x20 Deadlift 3x12 Jumping Jacks 3x12 Leg Press 3x12 Calf Raise 3x16	Decline bench press 3x10 Row 3x12 Rear delt raise 3x15 DB curl 3x12 Overhead tricep extension 3x12 Military press 3x10	REST
DAY 7	**DAY 8**	**DAY 9**
Incline press 3x16 Tricep dip 3x25 Pull-ups 3x12 Military press 3x15 Bent-over row 3x15 Push-ups 3x25	REST	Deadlift 3x10 Bench press 4x8 Deadlift 1x12 Squat 1x12 Deadlift 1x10 Squat 1x10 Deadlift 1x8 Squat 1x8 Deadlift 1x6 Squat 1x6
DAY 10	**DAY 11**	**DAY 12**
Bench press 3x10 DB incline press 3x12 Push-ups 3x12 DB press 3x12 DB fly 3x12 Machine shoulder press 3x10	REST	Lunges 3x30 Squats 3x10 Prisoner squat 3x15 Side lunge 3x30 Leg press 3x12 Calf raise 3x16

30-Day Full Body Program, cont'd.

DAY 13	DAY 14	DAY 15
Plank 3x1 min Bicycle crunches 3x30 Decline crunches 3x15 Hanging leg raise 3x15 Weighted v-ups 3x25 Stair climber 30 mins	REST	Leg press 3x10 Incline press 3x8 Low row 3x8 Squats 3x8 Machine shoulder press 3x10 Bent-over row 3x10
DAY 16	**DAY 17**	**DAY 18**
Reverse grip pull-up 3x20 Rear delt raise 3x10 Bent-over row 3x10 Pull-ups 3x12 Shoulder shrugs 3x15 Military press 3x10	Jumping jacks 3x50 High knees 3x50 Butt kicks 3x40 High kicks 3x40 Push-ups 3x25 Sprints 10x100 meters	REST
DAY 19	**DAY 20**	**DAY 21**
Lunges 3x20 Squats 3x20 Deadlift 3x10 Leg extension 3x20 Leg press 3x12 Calf raise 3x16	Planks 4x1 Min. Side planks 4x1 Min. Sit-ups 3x25 Reverse crunch 3x20 Russian twists 3x40 Jog 20 Min.	Decline bench press 3x12 DB fly 3x16 Shoulder shrugs 3x15 Deadlift 3x10 Bent-over row 3x10 DB incline press 3x12

30-Day Full Body Program, cont'd.

DAY 22	DAY 23	DAY 24
REST	Jumping jacks 3 x 50 High knees 3 x 50 Butt kicks 3 x 40 High kicks 3 x 40 Push-ups 3 x 25 Sprints 10 x 100 meters	Machine shoulder press 3 x 15 Front raise 3 x 15 Side raise 3 x 15 Seated DB press 3 x 10 Shoulder shrugs 3 x 10 Military press 3 x 10
DAY 25	**DAY 26**	**DAY 27**
REST	Squats 3 x 10 Leg extension 3 x 10 Front squats 3 x 10 Leg press 3 x 8 Calf raise 3 x 16 Hanging leg raise 3 x 15	Preacher curl 3 x 10 Tricep dips 3 x 10 Hammer curl 3 x 16 Overhead tricep extension 3 x 10 Seated isolated curl 3 x 15 Preacher curl 3 x 25
DAY 28	**DAY 29**	**DAY 30**
Side plank dips 3 x 30 Scissor dicks 3 x 30 Superman 3 x 16 V-ups 3 x 15 Oblique v-ups 3 x 15 (each side) Scissor kicks 3 x 30	REST	Bench press 4 x 10 Deadlift 3 x 10 Push-ups 3 x 20 DB press 3 x 8 Pull-ups 3 x Max Low row 3 x 16

PART 4: CREATING YOUR FITNESS PLAN

Now that you know what's needed for a healthy lifestyle, create your own fitness plan that caters to your body and goals.

Your Goal

What is your goal?

....

....

....

When will you accomplish your goal?

....

....

What activities and eating habits will help you accomplish your goal?

....

....

....

Your Motto

Use your goals to create a personal motto. This slogan will remind you of why you began your journey, and motivate you even when you want to give up.

....

....

....

Your Schedule

Remember, take one day at a time. That way you won't overwhelm yourself!

Use the following legend as you plan your own Weekly Schedule:

TIME OR PERIOD	Sun	Mon	Tues	Wed	Thu	Fri	Sat
6 am	S	F	F	F	F	F	S
7 am	S	M	M	M	M	M	S
8 am	S	C	WO	C	WO	C	F

Legend

EC = Extracurricular activities

C = Class or lab

F = Free time

M = Meal

WO = Workout

W = Work

HW = Homework or study group

S = Sleep

Week Number

TIME OR PERIOD	Sun	Mon	Tues	Wed	Thu	Fri	Sat

DOWNLOAD PDF FORMS AT ARIELLETOLBERT.COM

Week Number ☐

TIME OR PERIOD	Sun	Mon	Tues	Wed	Thu	Fri	Sat

Week Number

TIME OR PERIOD	Sun	Mon	Tues	Wed	Thu	Fri	Sat

Week Number ☐

TIME OR PERIOD	Sun	Mon	Tues	Wed	Thu	Fri	Sat

Your Workout

Consistency is key—if you miss a workout, just get back on track the next day!

EX = Exercise SxR = Sets x Reps	SUN	MON	TUE	WED
EX				
S x R				
EX				
S x R				
EX				
S x R				
EX				
S x R				
EX				
S x R				
EX				
S x R				
EX				
S x R				
EX				
S x R				
EX				
S x R				
EX				
S x R				

DOWNLOAD PDF FORMS AT ARIELLETOLBERT.COM

Your Workout

EX = Exercise SxR = Sets x Reps	THU	FRI	SAT
EX			
S x R			
EX			
S x R			
EX			
S x R			
EX			
S x R			
EX			
S x R			
EX			
S x R			
EX			
S x R			
EX			
S x R			
EX			
S x R			
EX			
S x R			
EX			
S x R			

Your Workout Log

EX = Exercise SxR = Sets x Reps	DATE	DATE	DATE
EX			
WEIGHT			
S x R			
EX			
WEIGHT			
S x R			
EX			
WEIGHT			
S x R			
EX			
WEIGHT			
S x R			
EX			
WEIGHT			
S x R			
EX			
WEIGHT			
S x R			
EX			
WEIGHT			
S x R			

Your Workout Log

EX = Exercise SxR = Sets x Reps	DATE	DATE	DATE
EX			
WEIGHT			
S x R			
EX			
WEIGHT			
S x R			
EX			
WEIGHT			
S x R			
EX			
WEIGHT			
S x R			
EX			
WEIGHT			
S x R			
EX			
WEIGHT			
S x R			
EX			
WEIGHT			
S x R			

Becoming a Better YOU

It is easy to lose track of your nutrition and fitness goals. If that time comes, you must remember why you started this journey and the benefits a healthy lifestyle will have on your life.

If you find yourself needing more motivation, grab a friend and bring them on this journey with you. Having a friend with you will remind you of your motto, and constantly motivate you to push yourself to your limit.

It is always fun to work out with a partner, but understand that what your partner does will not affect you. Every body is different and reacts to exercises differently.

Although it is fun to work out and set goals with a partner, remember the goals you want to accomplish will solely depend on you and how much time and effort you invest in yourself.

This is your guide to eating healthy, managing your time, working out, and not gaining the "Freshman 15."

This journey is **your** journey—don't let anyone or anything stop you from reaching your goals!

EXERCISE GALLERY

Ab Rollout

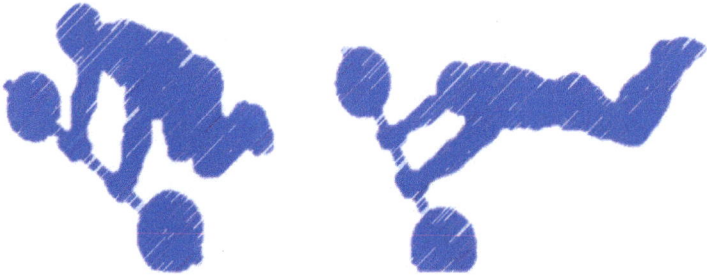

Alternating Fast Feet

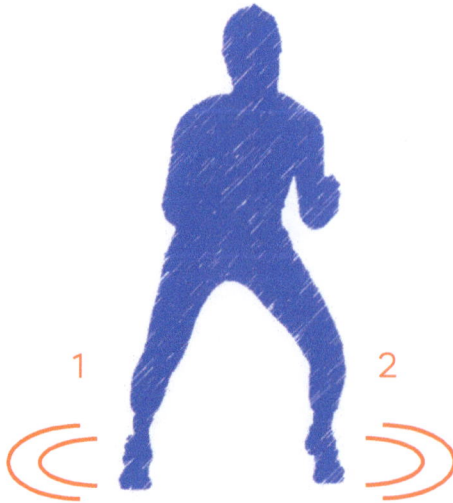

Alternating Split Jump

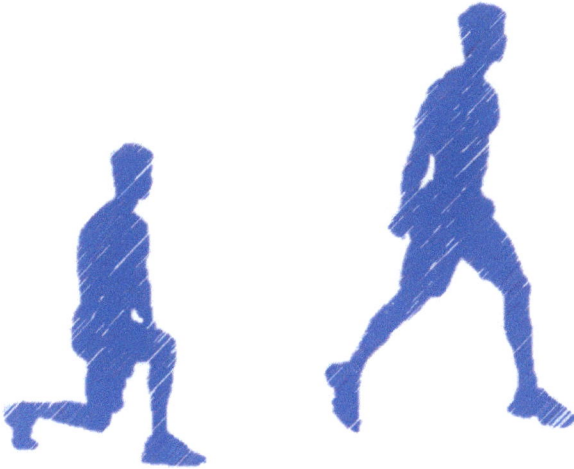

Alternating Step-Up Jump

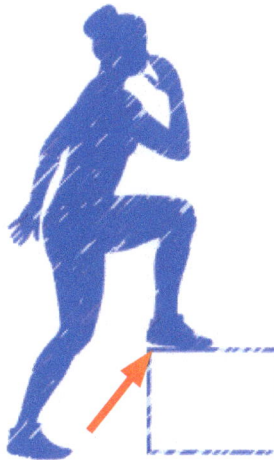

Ball Leg Curl

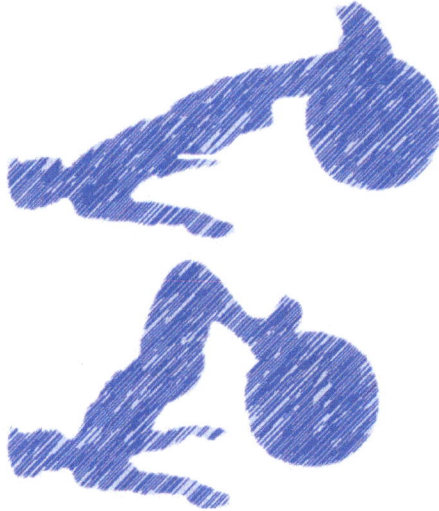

Bench / DB Press

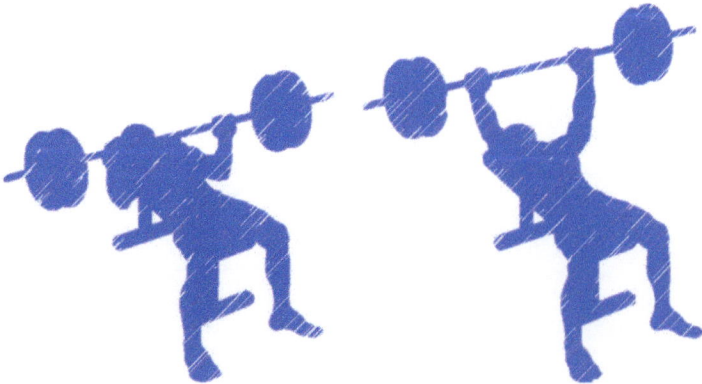

Bent Over Row

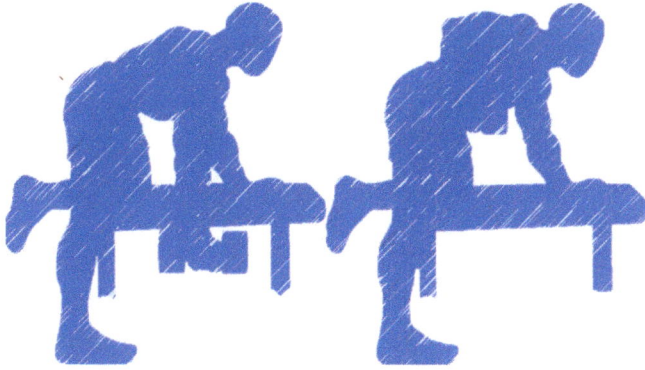

Bicycle Crunch

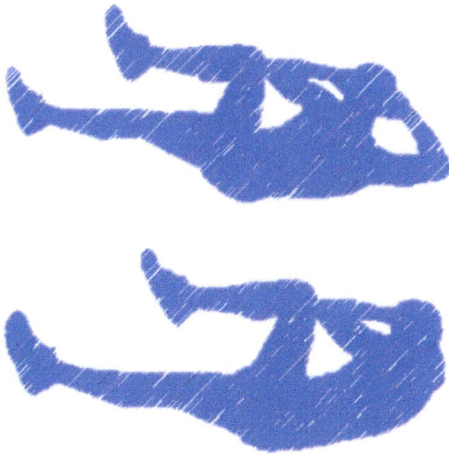

Cable Crunches

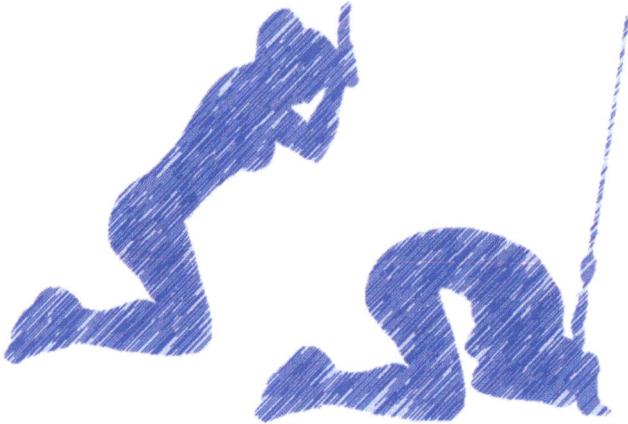

Blast-Off Pushup

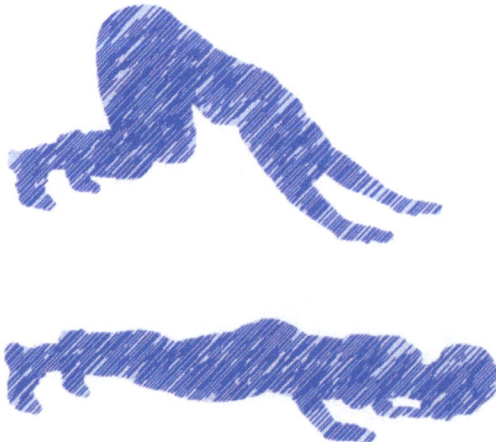

Box Squat Jump

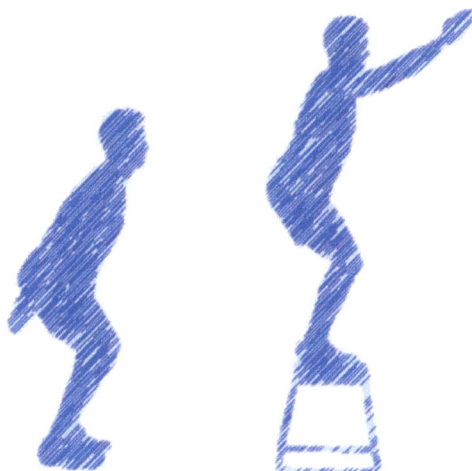

Break Dancer

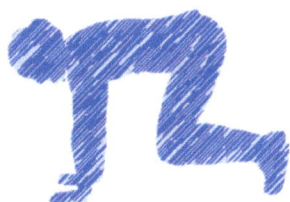

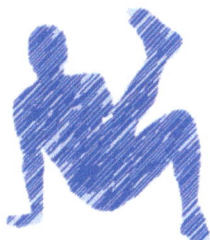

Bridges

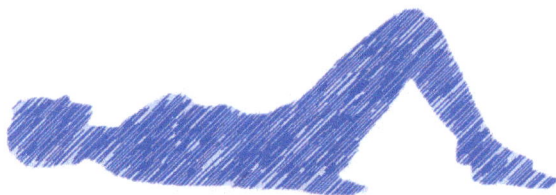

Burpees

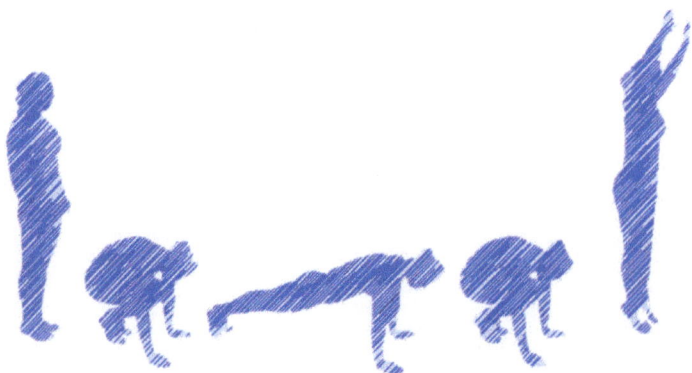

Butt Kicks

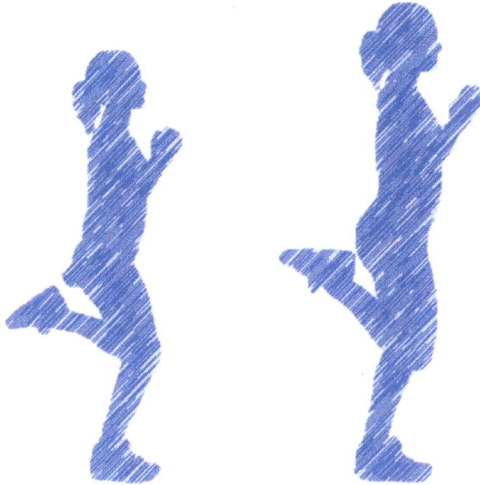

Calf Raise

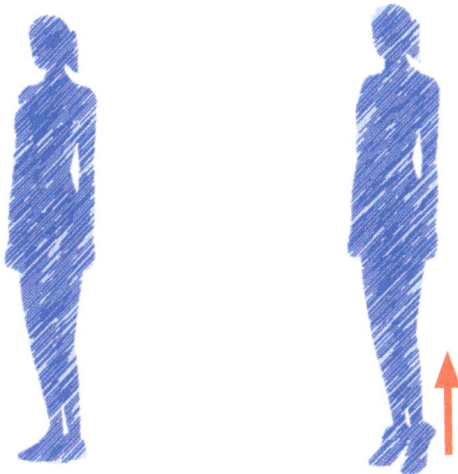

Chin Up

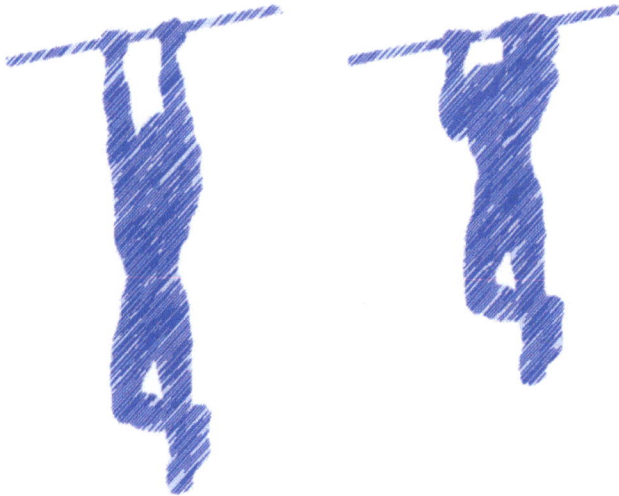

Crab Touch

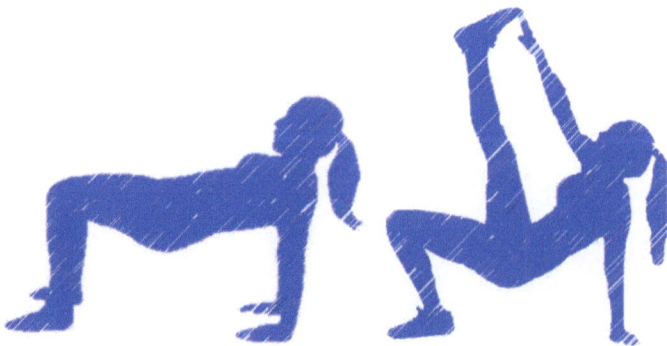

Cross-Body Jumping Jack

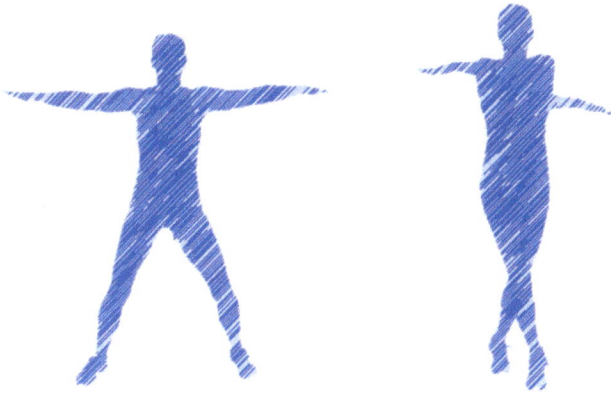

Deadlift

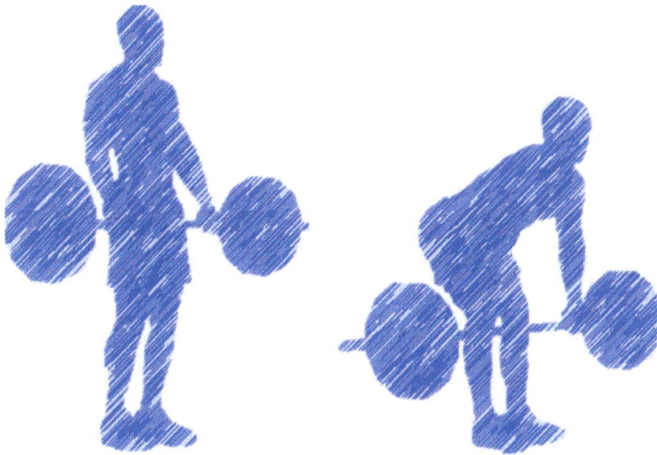

Decline Bench Press

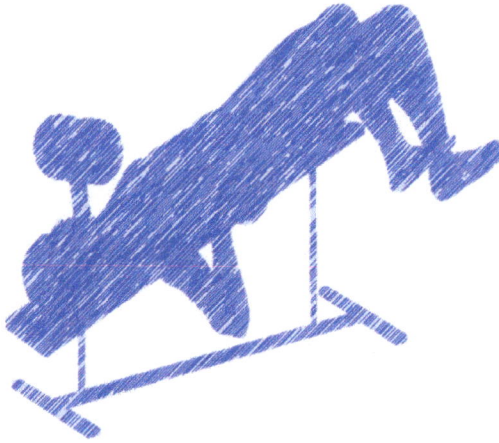

Decline Crunches

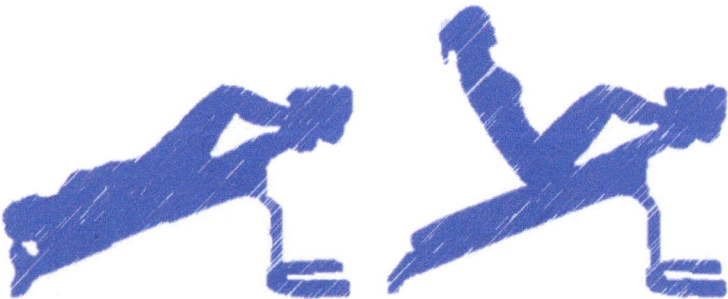

Diagonal Mountain Climber (knee to elbow)

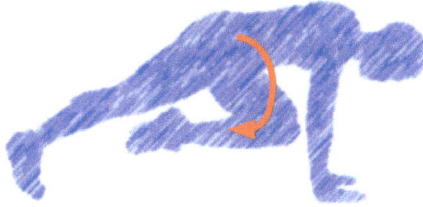

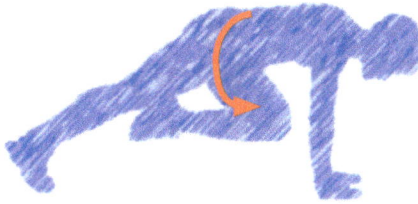

Donkey Kick

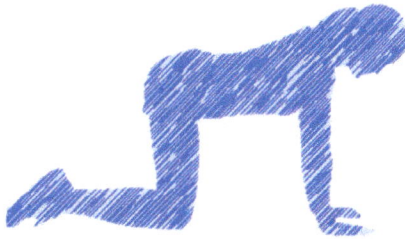

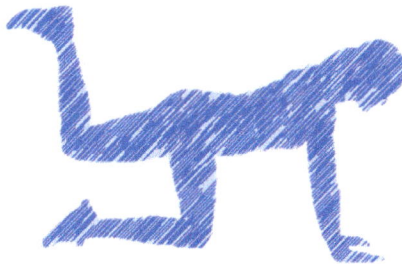

Double Fast Feet

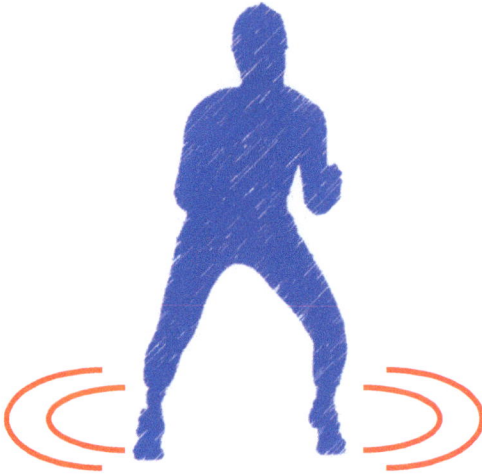

Drop Squat

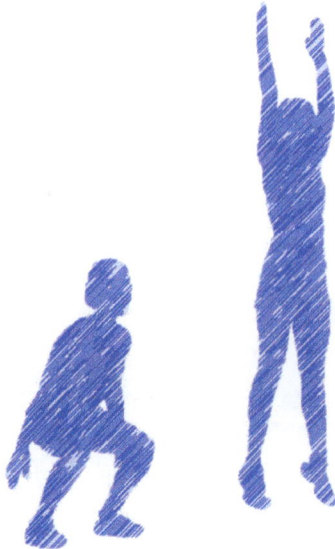

Drop Step Back Squat

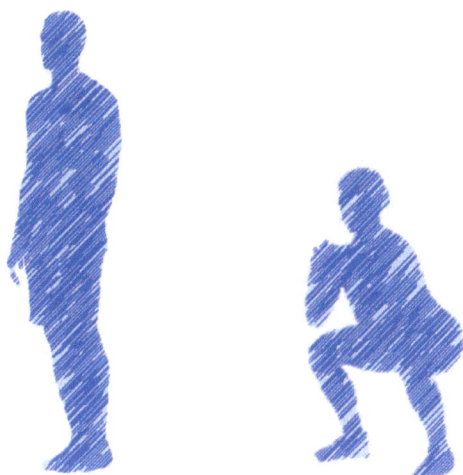

Dumbbell (DB) Curl

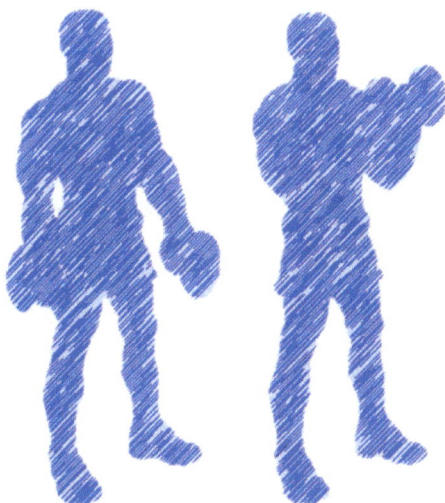

Dumbbell (DB) Curl & Press

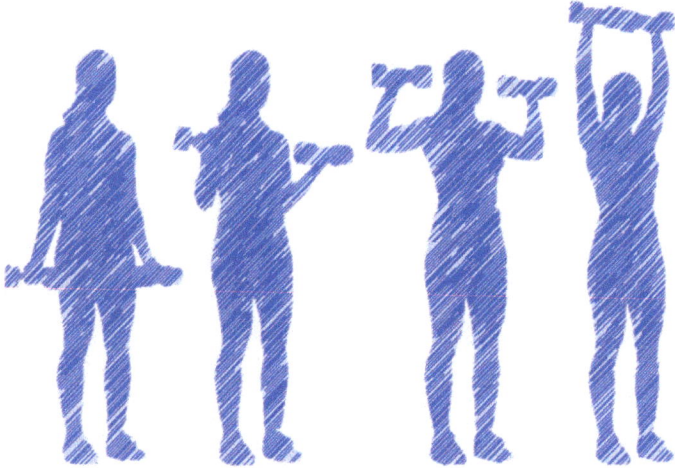

Dumbbell (DB) Fly

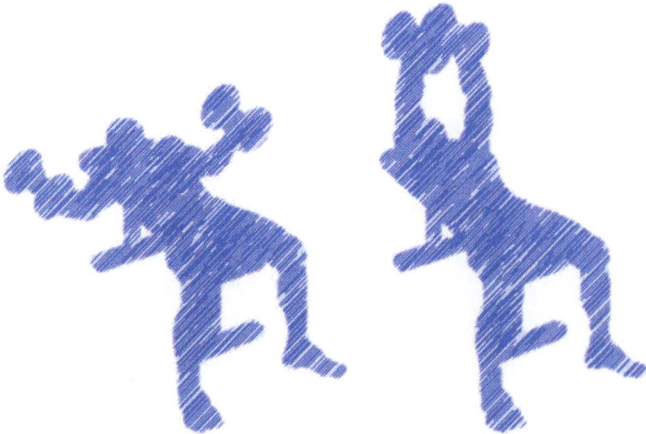

Dumbbell (DB) Incline Press

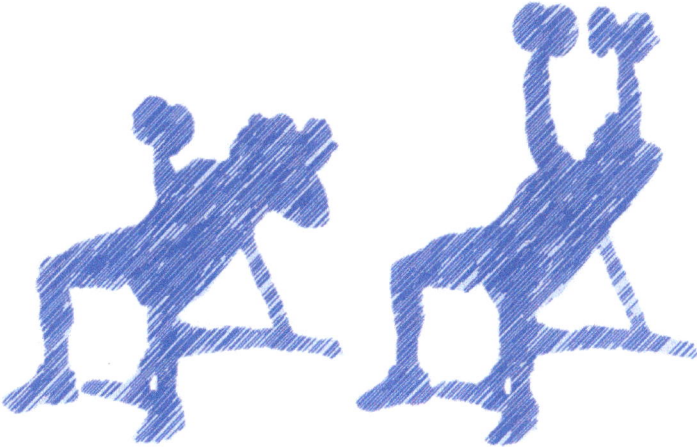

Dumbbell (DB) Side Raise

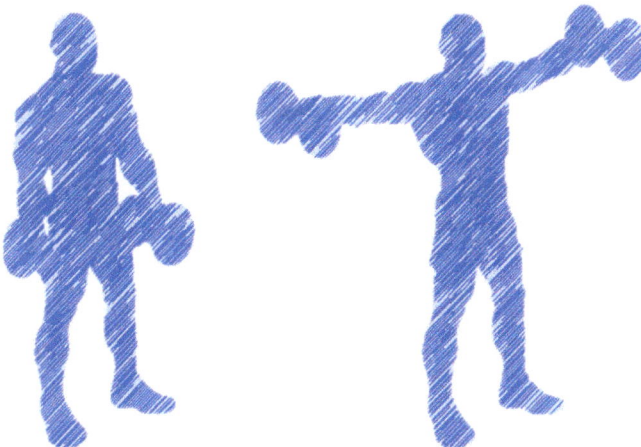

Dumbbell (DB) Split Squat

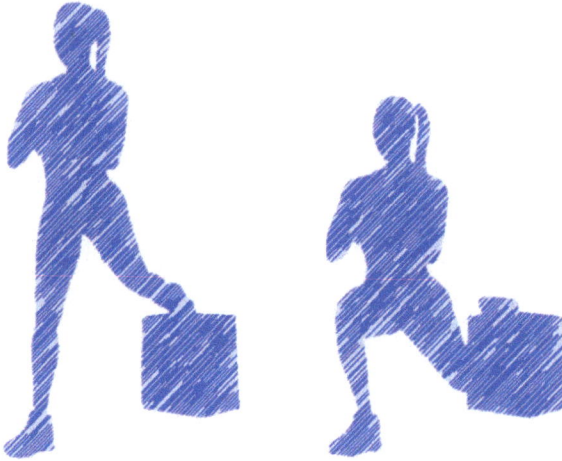

Face Melter Step-Ups

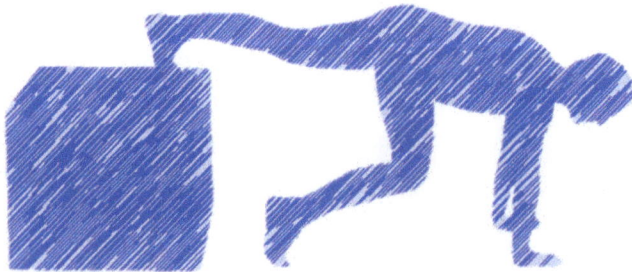

Fast Feet On Hands

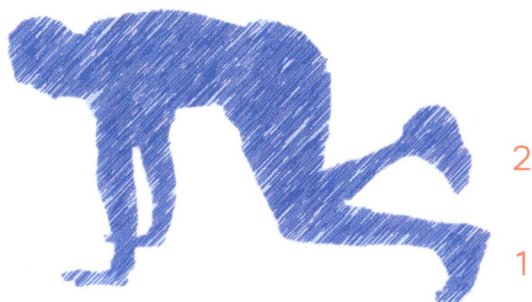

2

1

Floor Touches

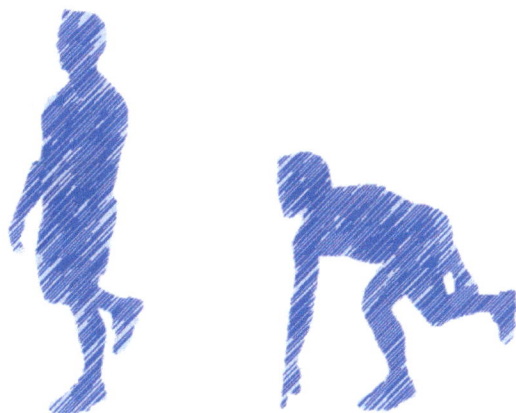

Flutter Kicks

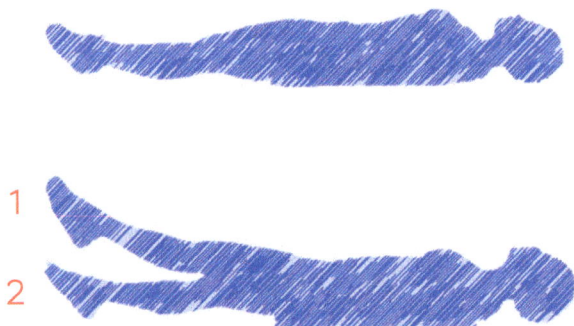

Front Raise

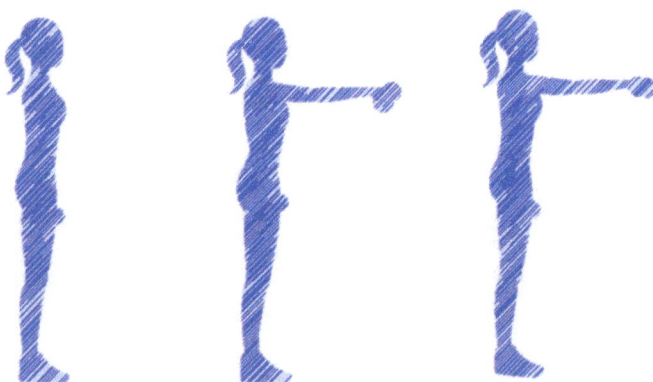

Front-to-Back Hop

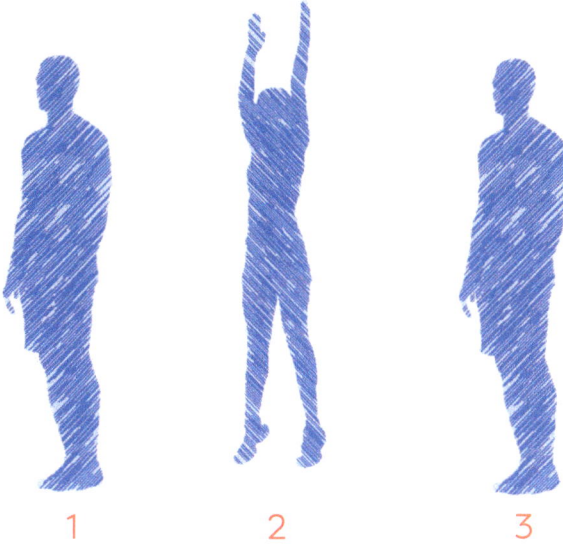

1   2   3

Front Squats

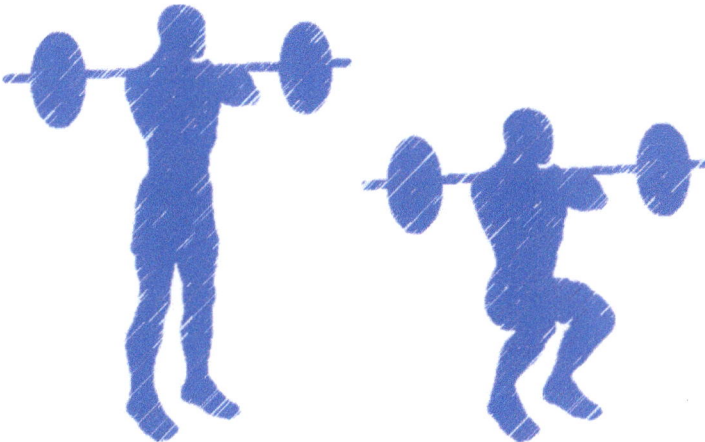

Halo Slam

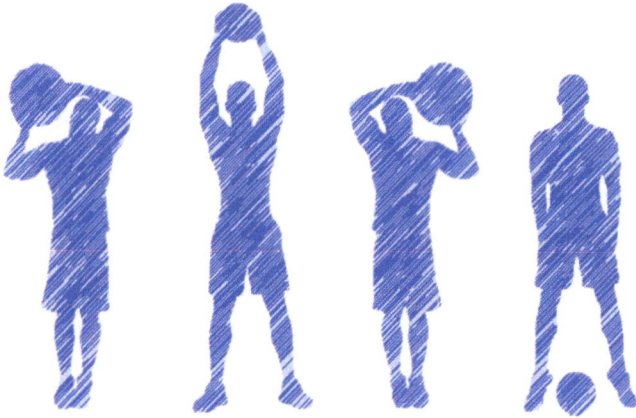

Hammer Curl

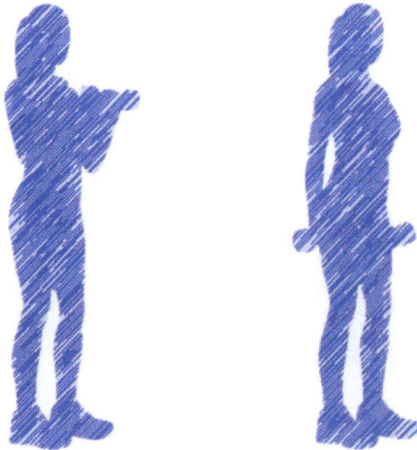

Hanging Leg Raise

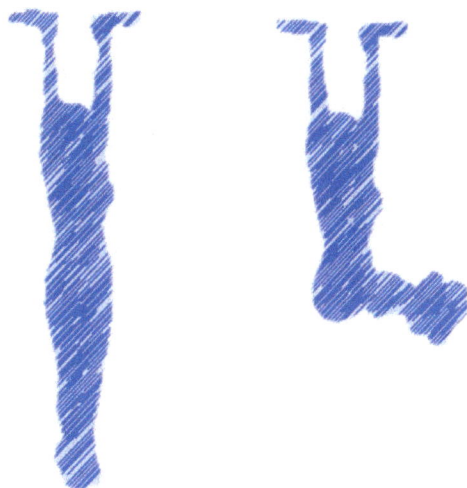

High Kicks

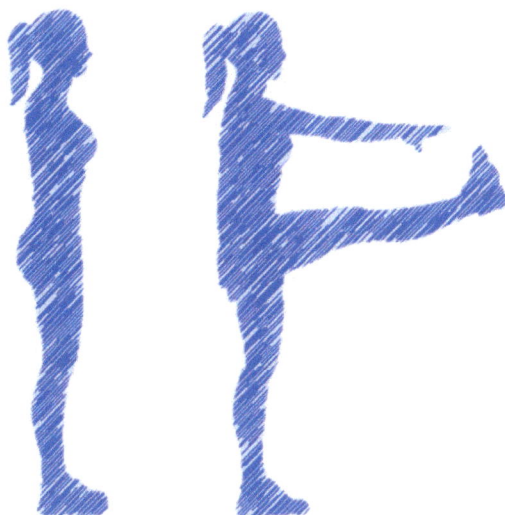

High-Knee Run

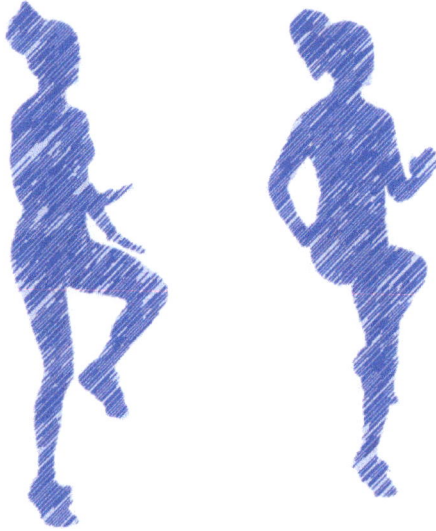

In-And-Out Squat Jacks

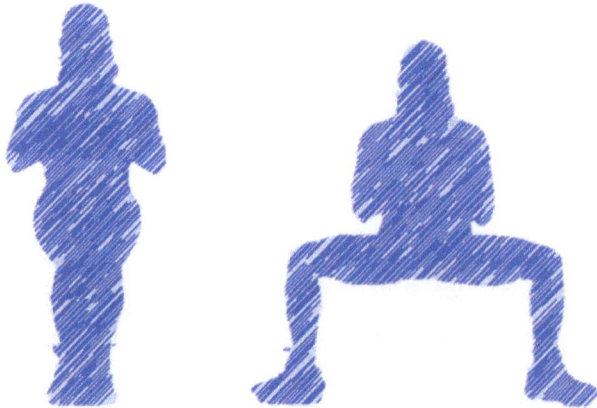

Inverted Row

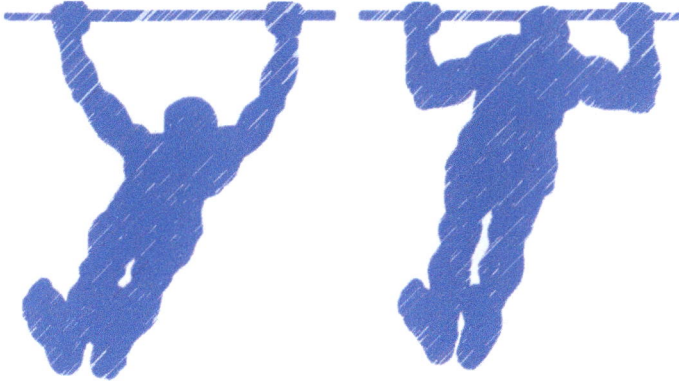

Jumping Jacks

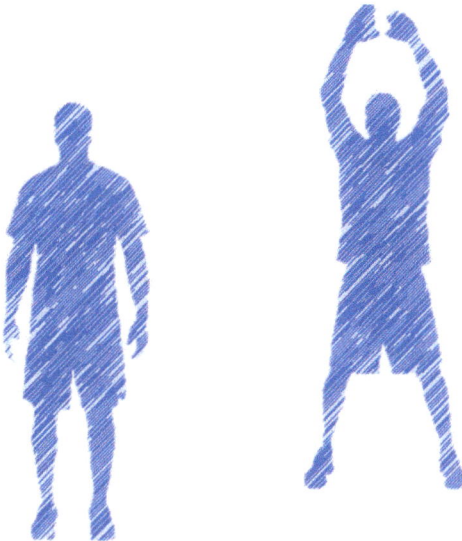

Jumping Mountain Climber

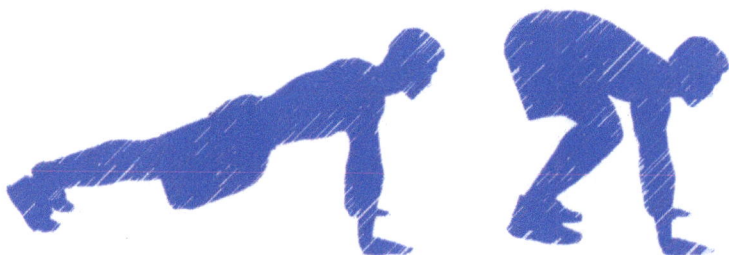

Karaoke

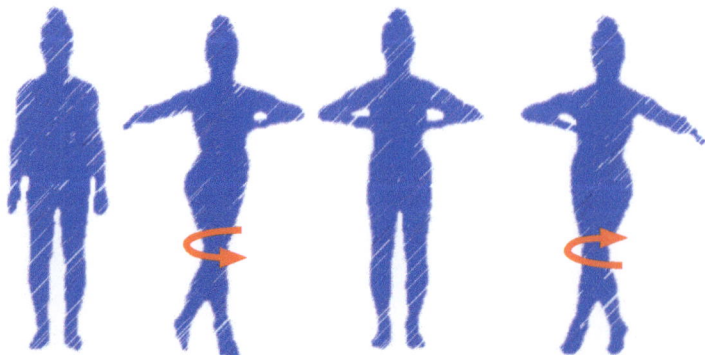

Lateral 3-Step

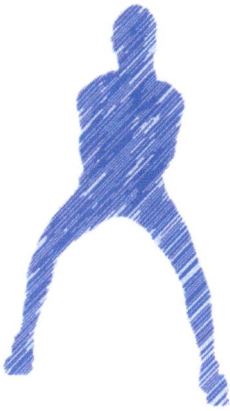 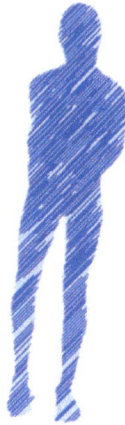 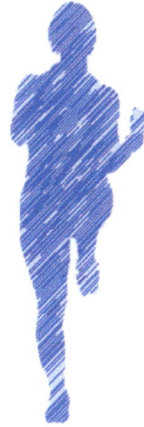

1   2   3

Leg Extensions

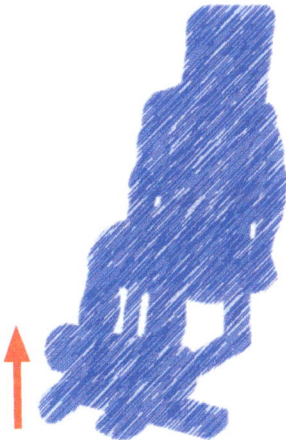 

Leg Press

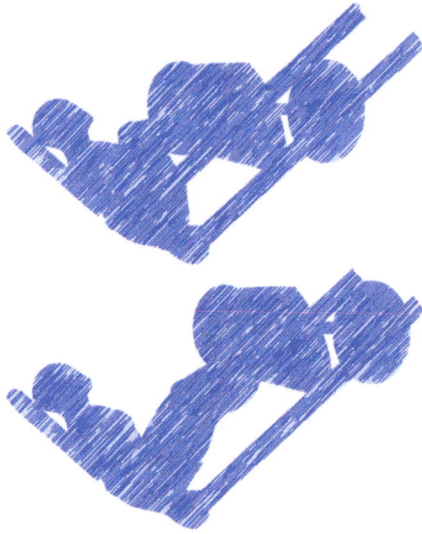

Leg Raises & Spreads

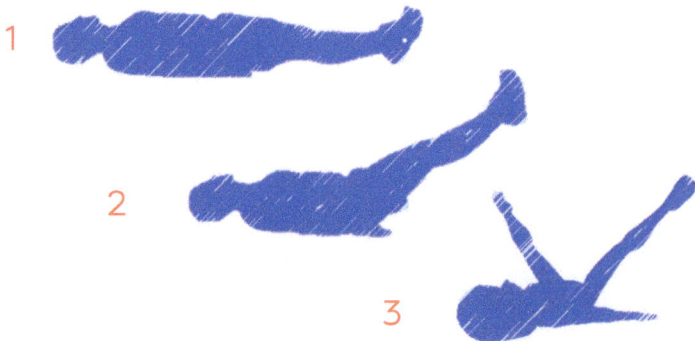

Long Jump & 3 Backward Hops

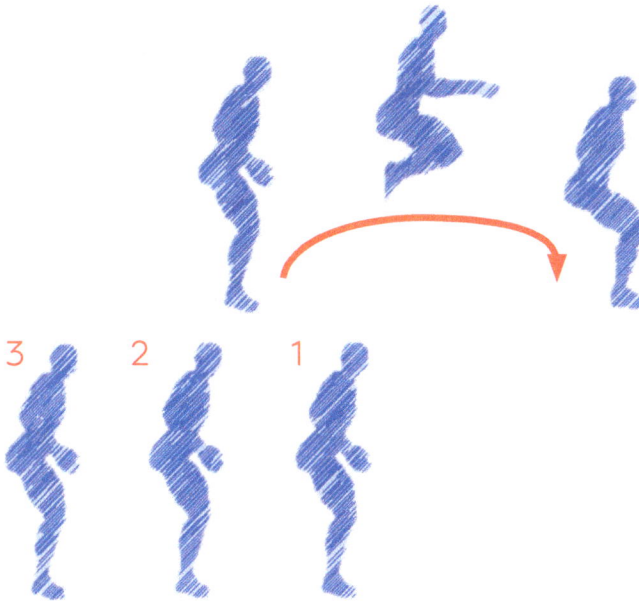

Low Box Lateral Runner

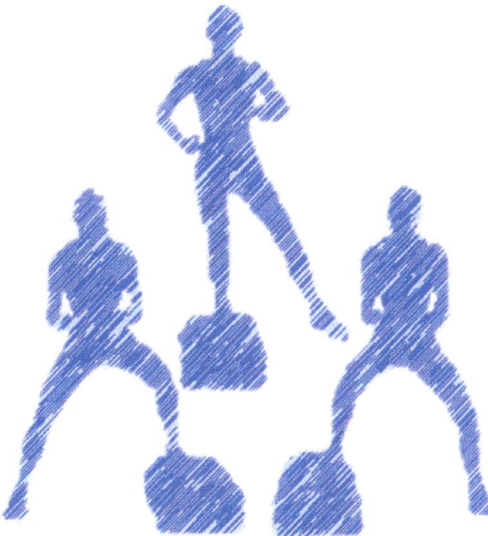

Low Box Runner

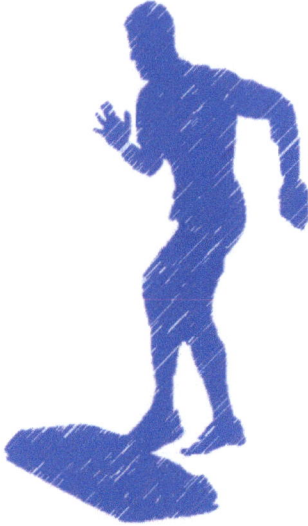

Low Rotational Chop

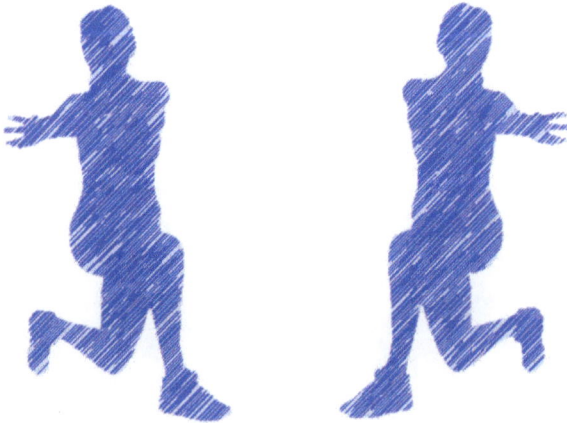

Low Row

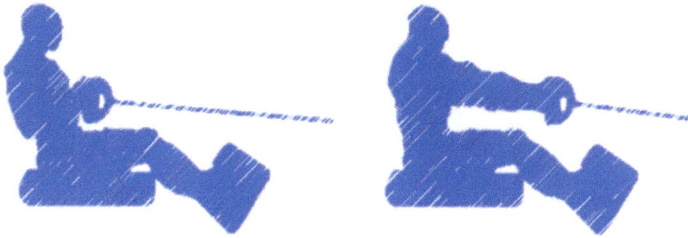

Low-Jumping Mountain Climber

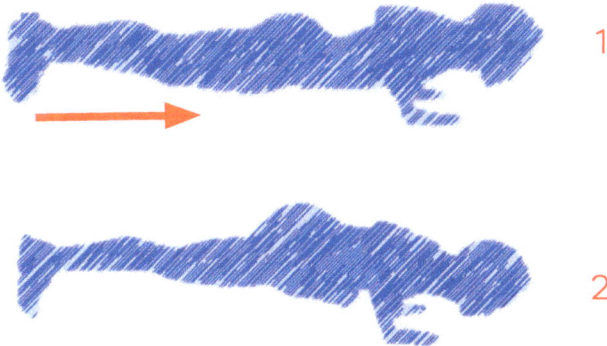

1

2

Lunges

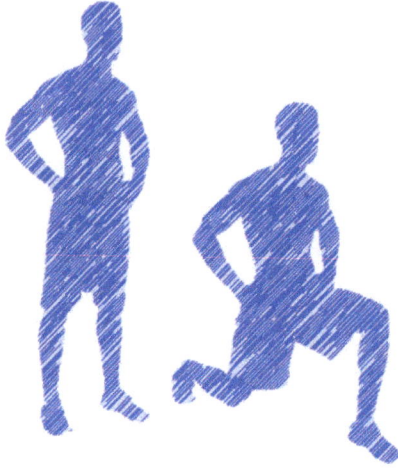

Lunge Runner

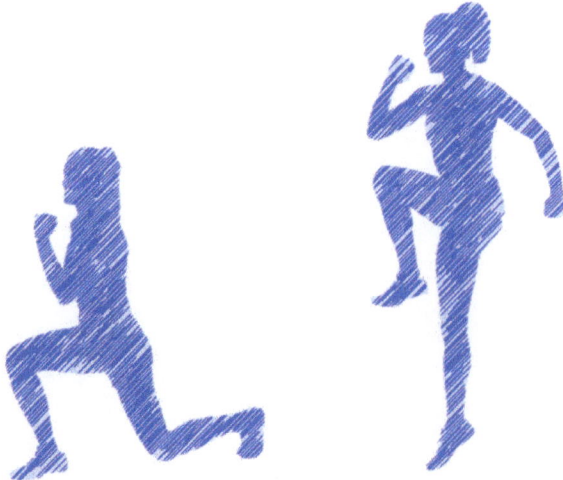

Machine Shoulder Press

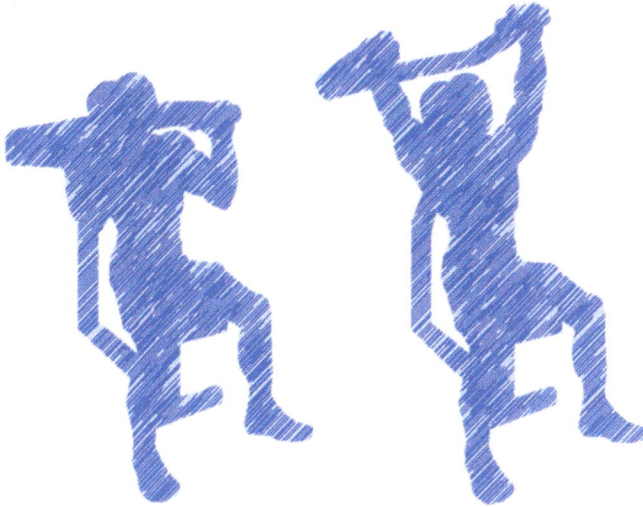

Military Press

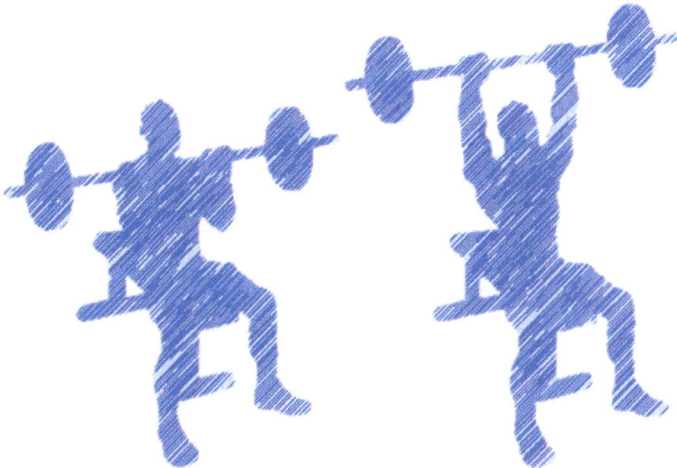

Mountain Climbers

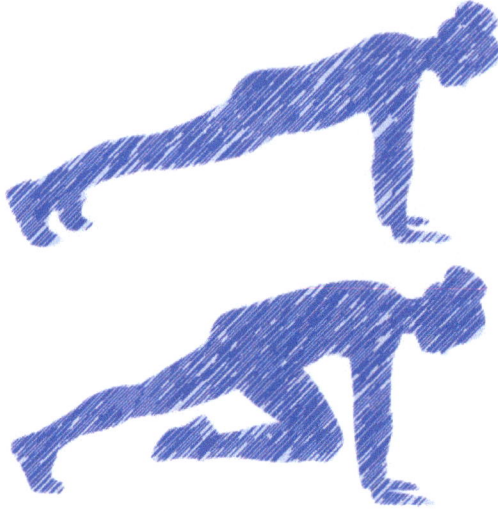

Oblique V-Ups

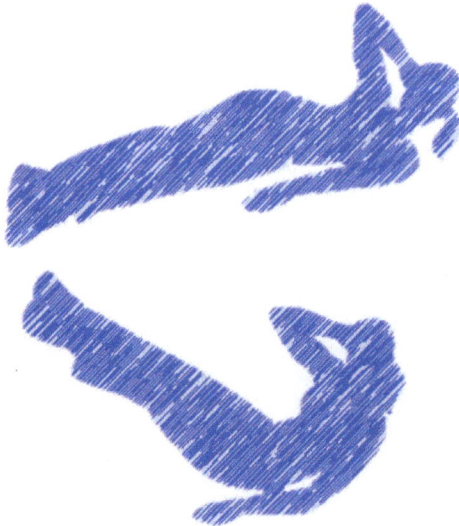

Overhead Tricep Extension

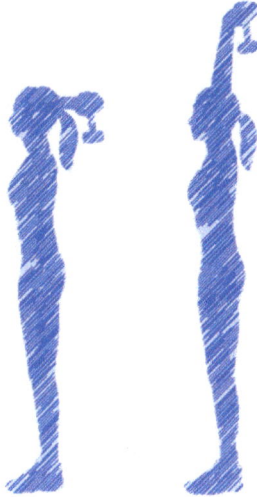

Planks

Plank Elbow Tap

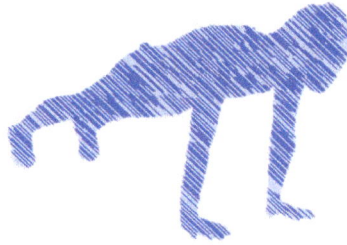

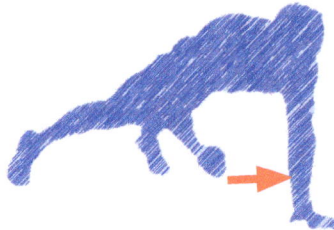

Plank Hand Tap

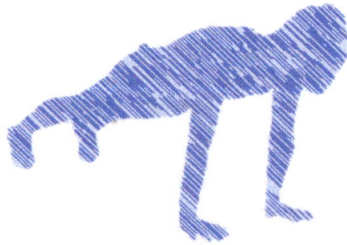

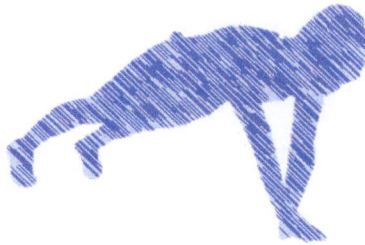

Plank Hip Tap

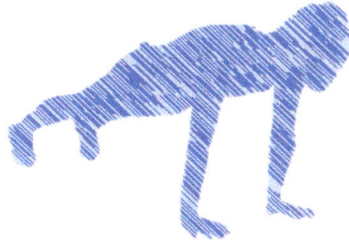

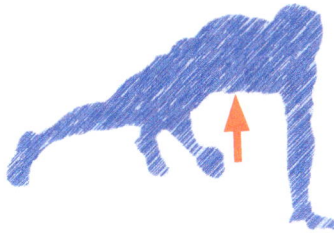

Plank Jacks

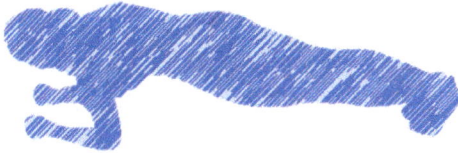

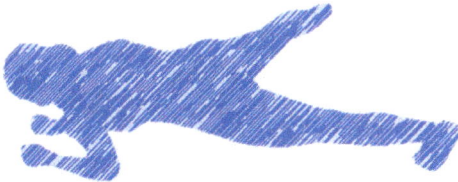

Plank Knee Tap

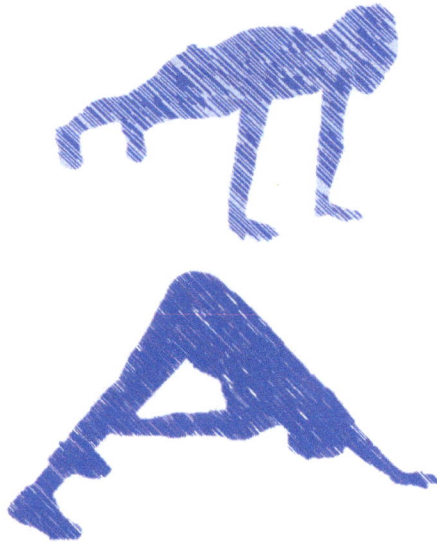

Plank Row

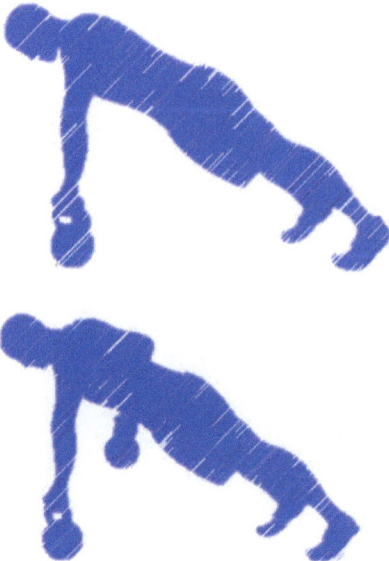

Plank Shoulder Tap

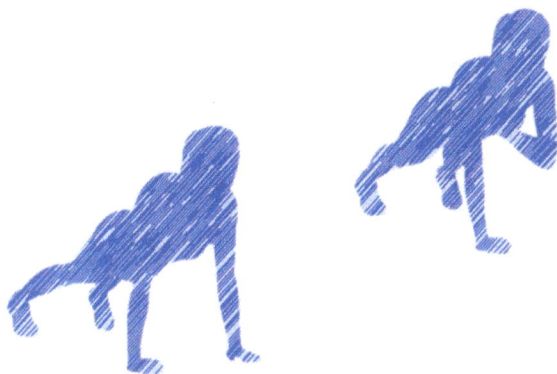

Plank Speed Reach

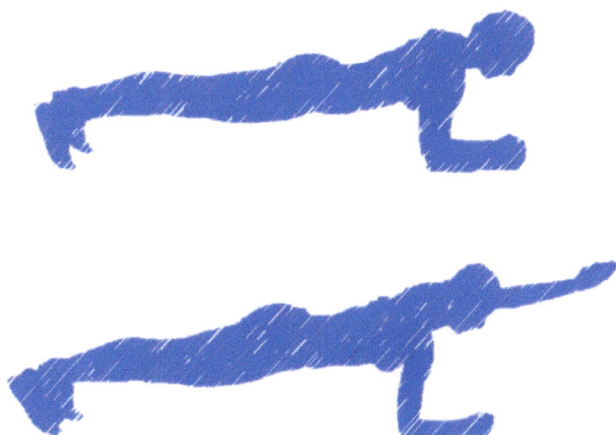

Plank Toe Tap

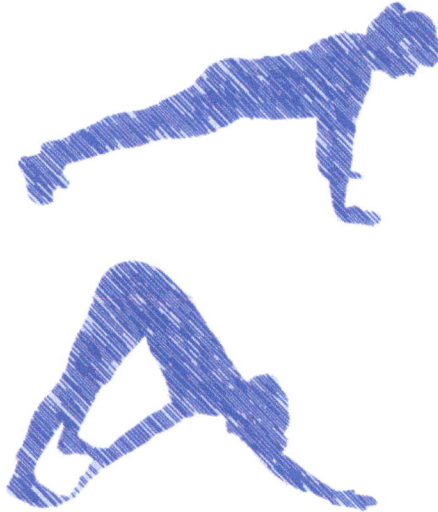

Plyo Alternating Single-Leg Hip Thrusts

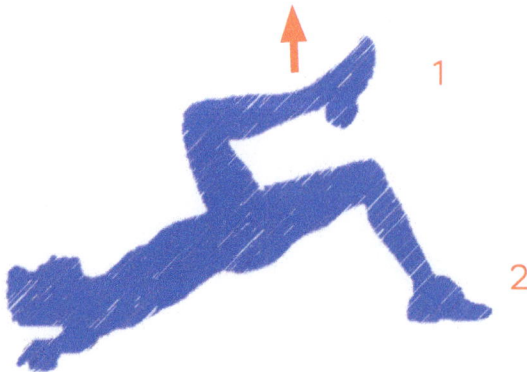

1

2

Plyo Clap Push-Up

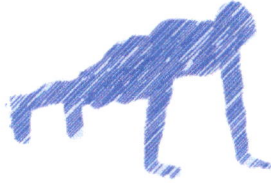

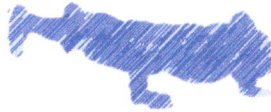

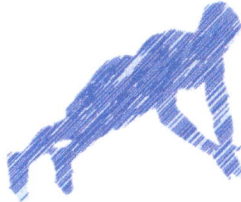

Plyo Single-Leg Hip Thrust

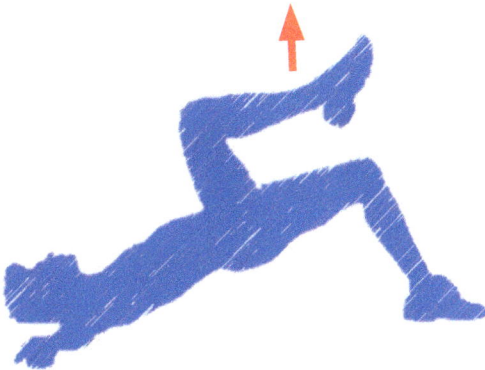

Pogo Jump

Power Skip

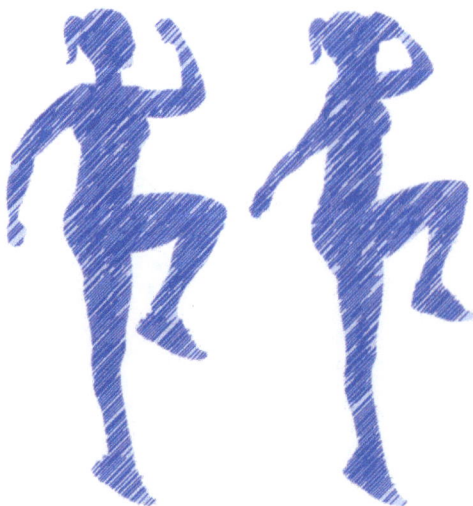

Preacher Curl

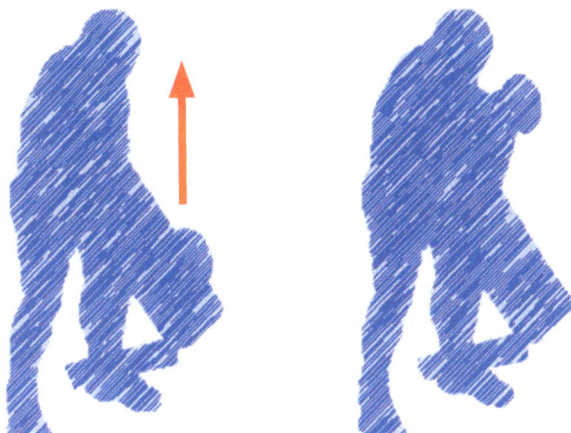

Predator Jack

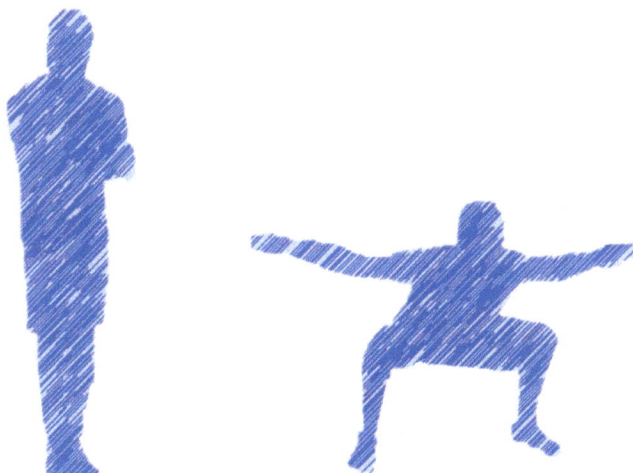

Prisoner Squat

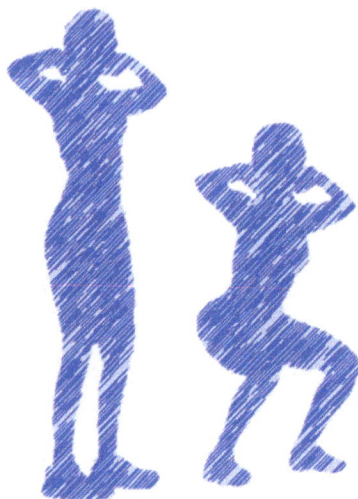

Pull-Ups

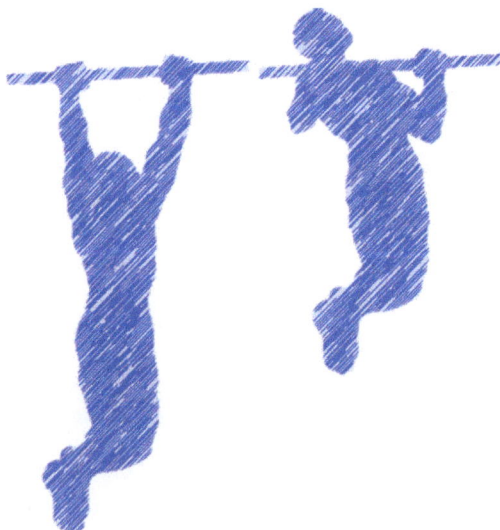

Pull-Downs

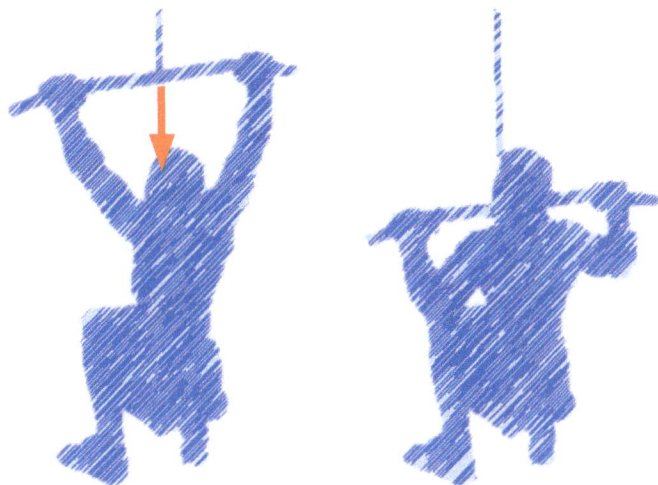

Pulse Squats

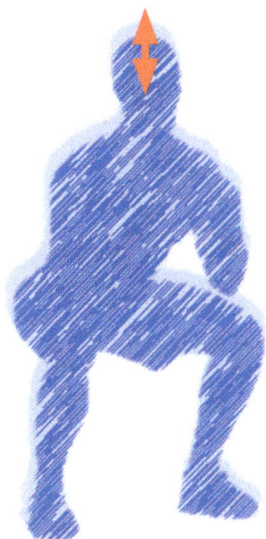

Punch

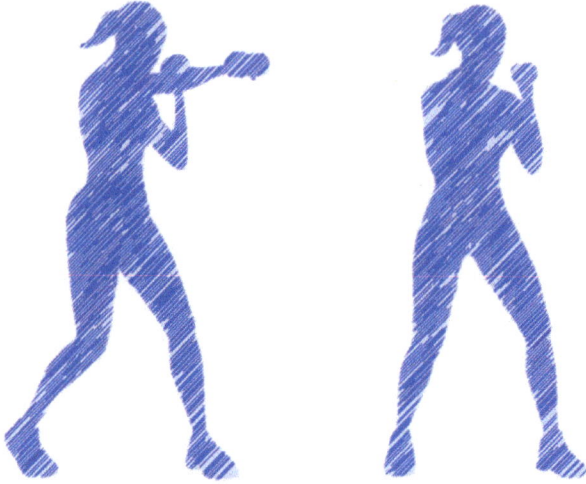

Push-Ups

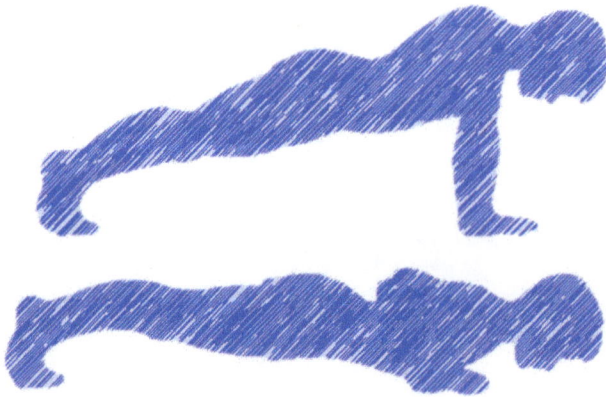

Push-Up Jack

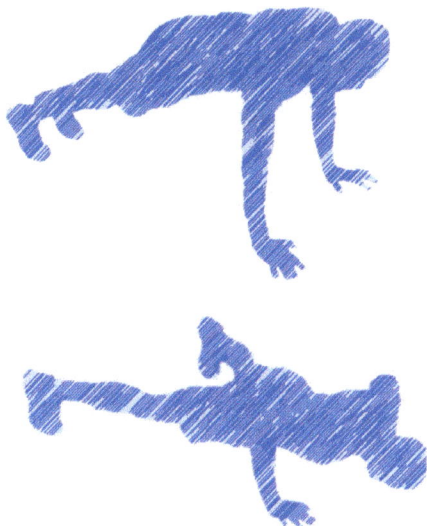

Quad Push-Up

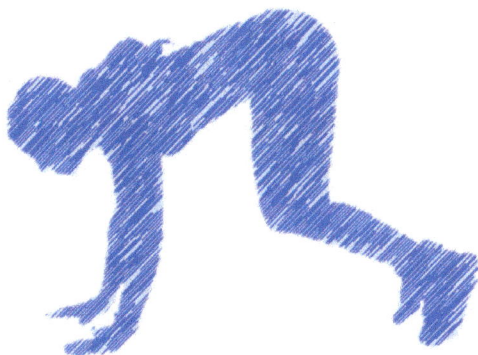

Rear Delt Raise

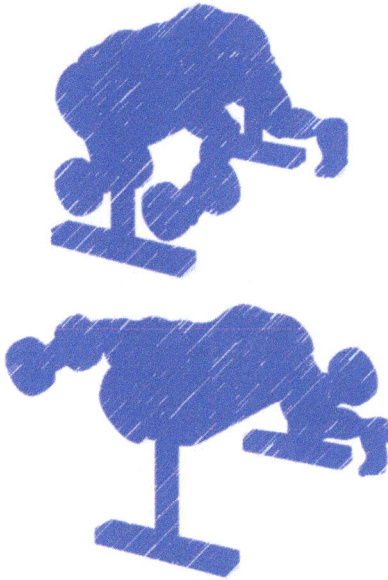

Reverse Crunch

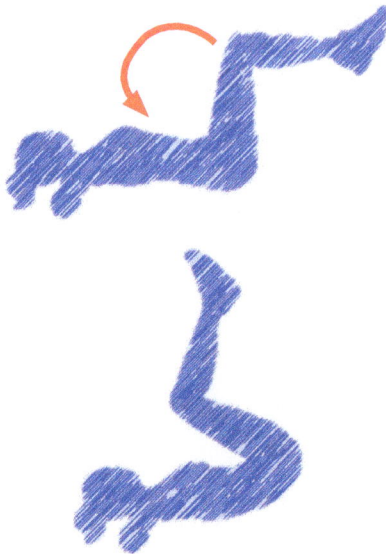

Reverse Grip Pull-Up

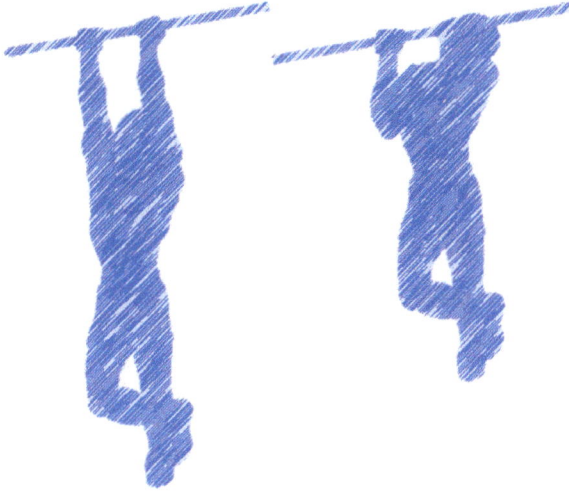

Rolling Squat Jump

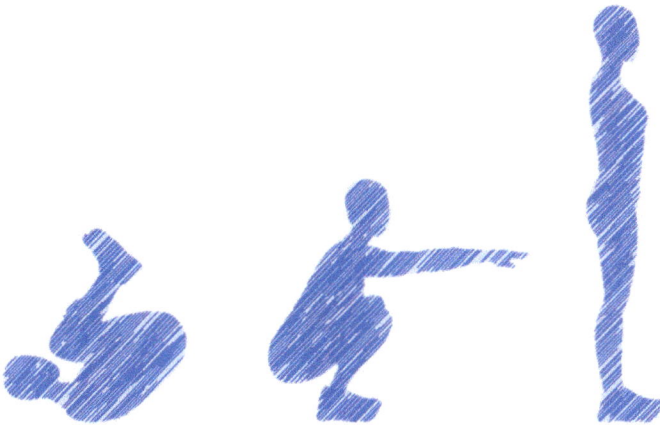

Rotational Chop

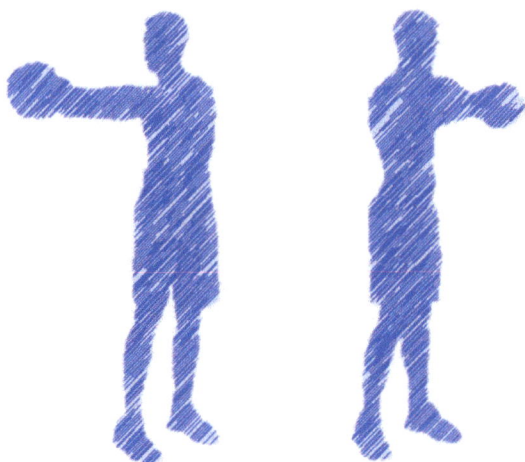

Russian Twist

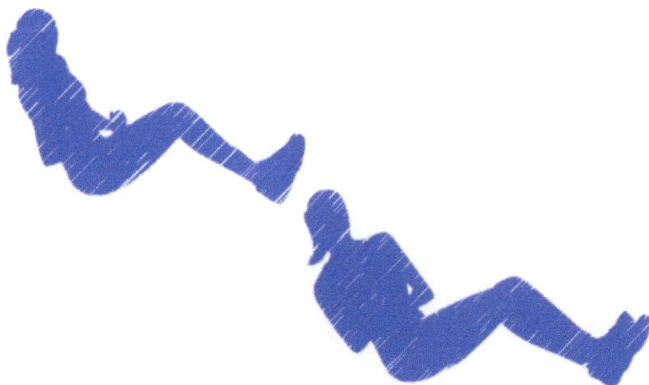

Scissor Kicks

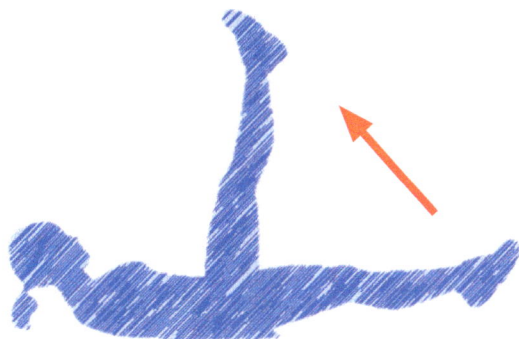

Seal Jack

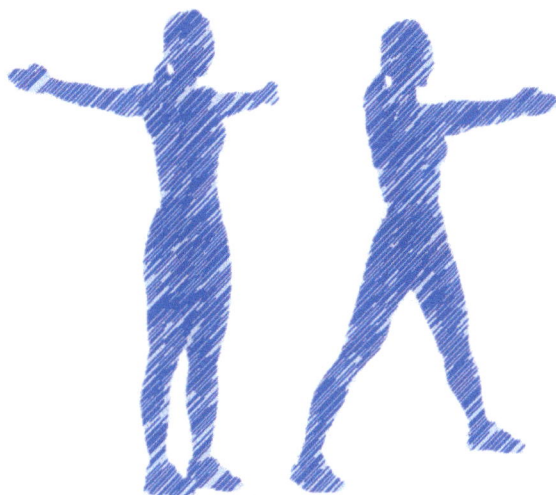

Seated Dumbbell (DB) Press

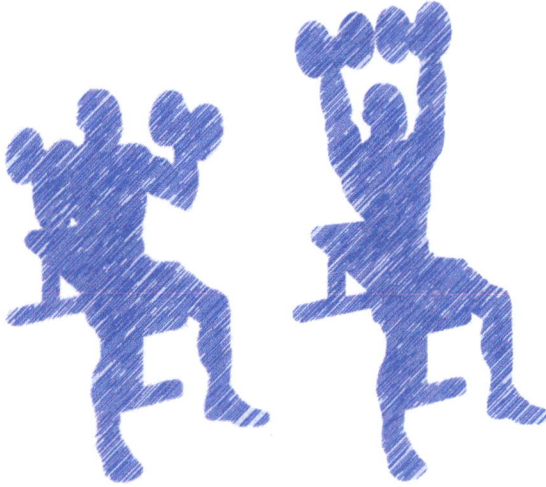

Seated Isolated Curl

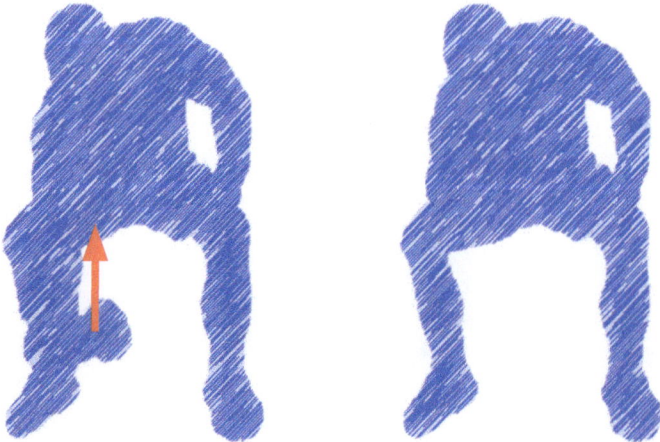

Shuffle In Place

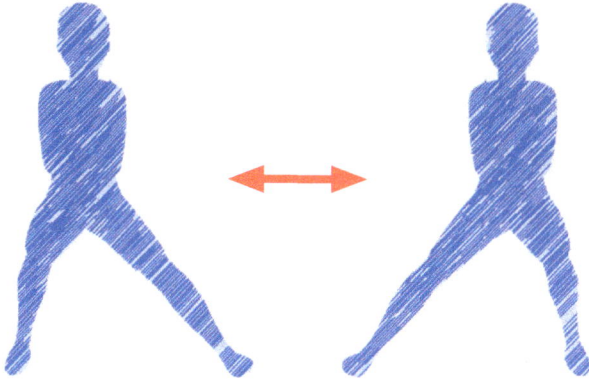

Shrugs

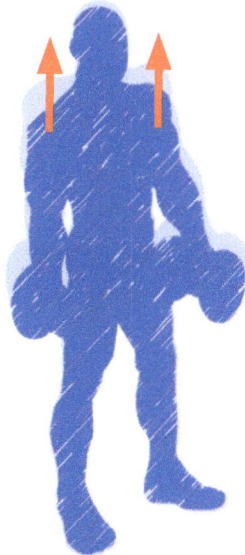

Side Lunges

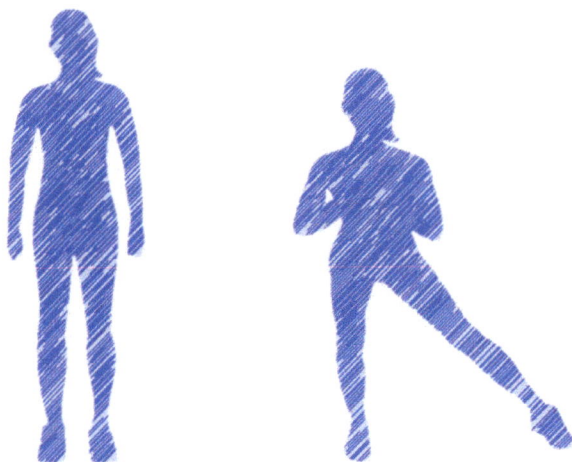

Side Plank

Side Plank Dips

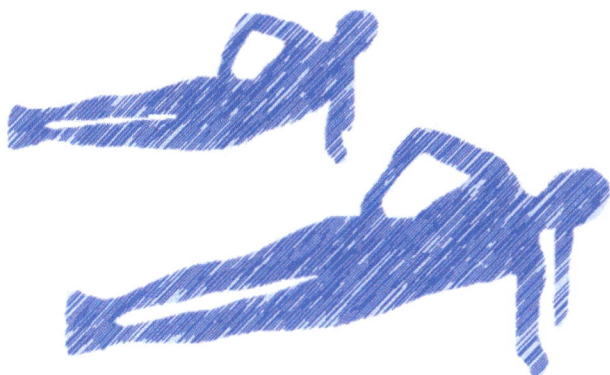

Side-To-Side Hop

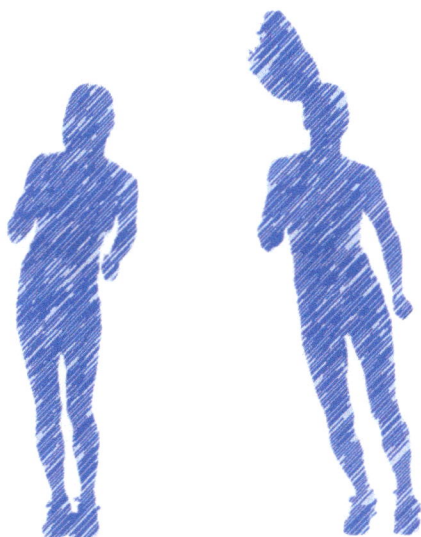

Side-To-Side Mountain Climber

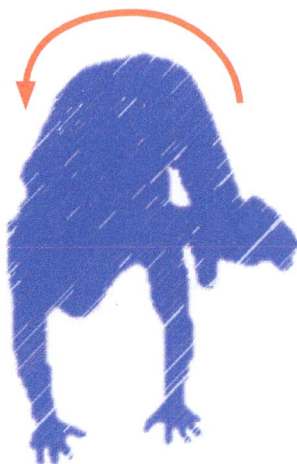

Single-Leg Pogo Jump

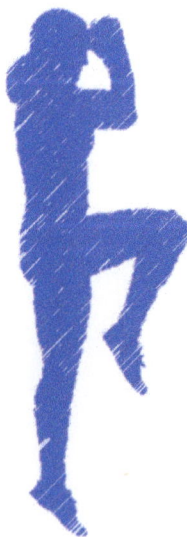

Single-Leg Swing

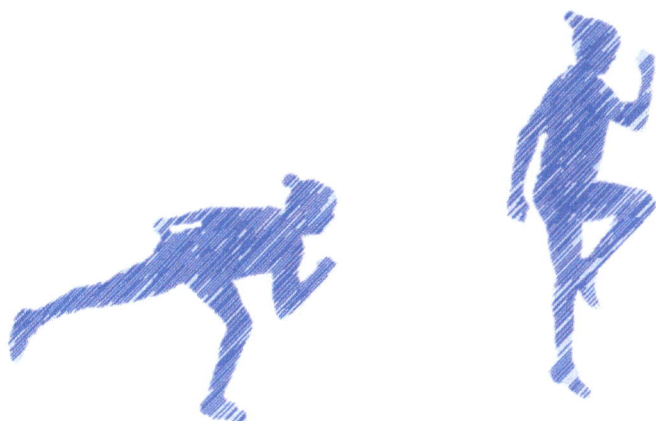

Sit-Ups

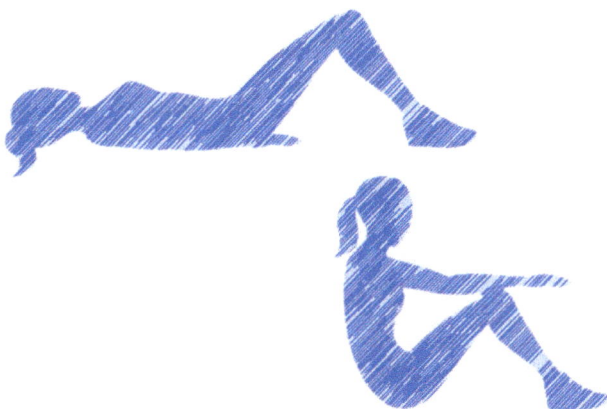

Skier Swing

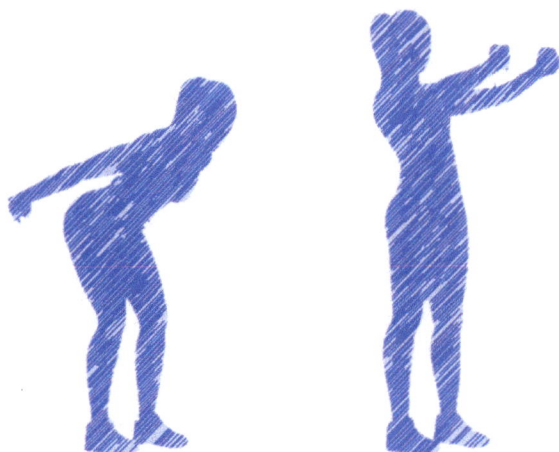

Slam

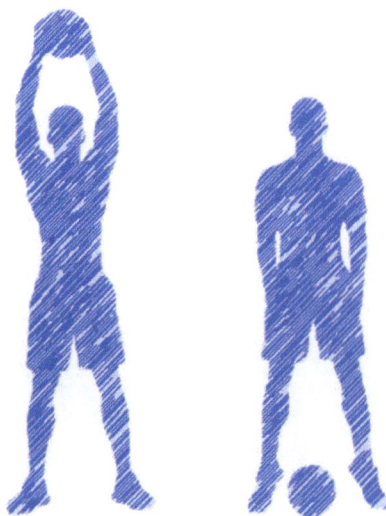

Speed Walkout

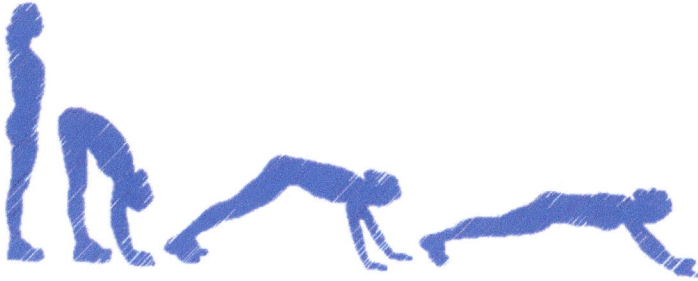

Spider Mountain Climber

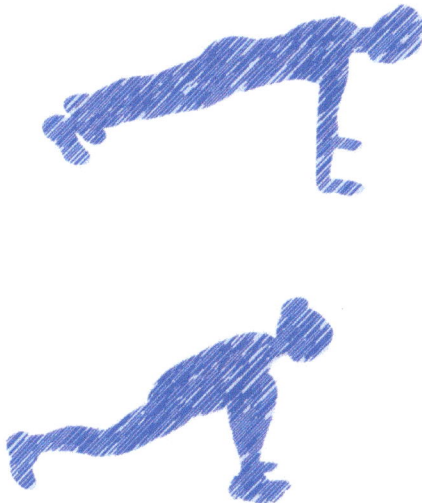

Sprinter Skip

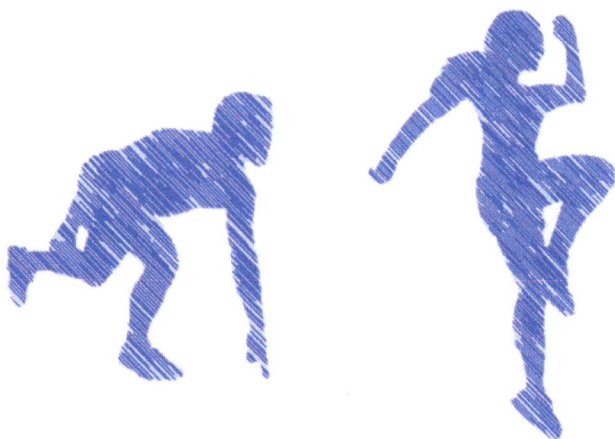

Sprinter Step

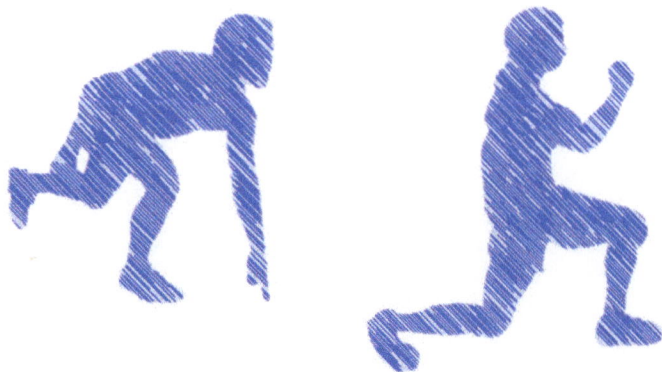

Squats

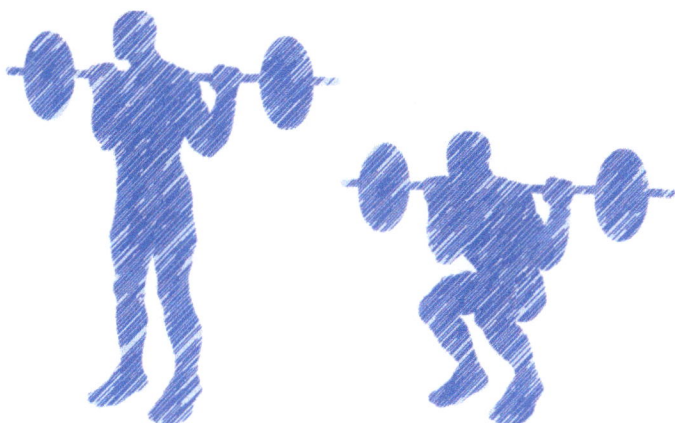

Squat Hold

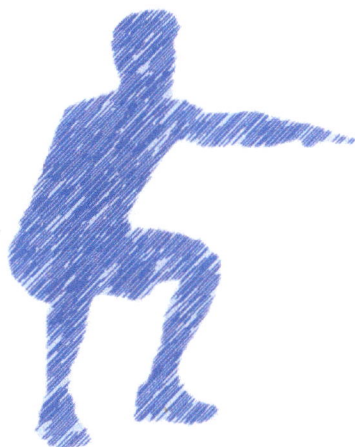

Squat With Leg Raise

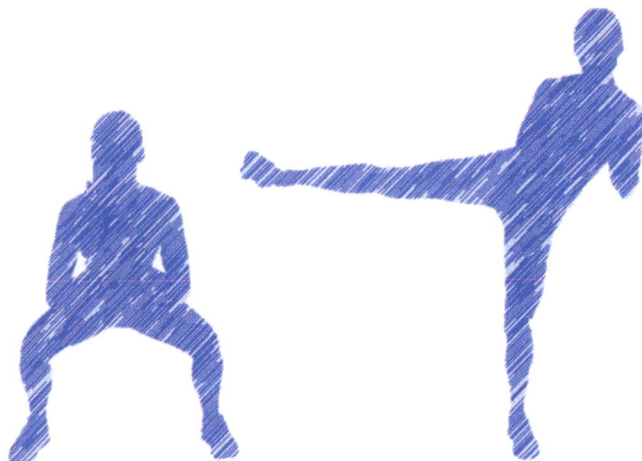

Squat Walk

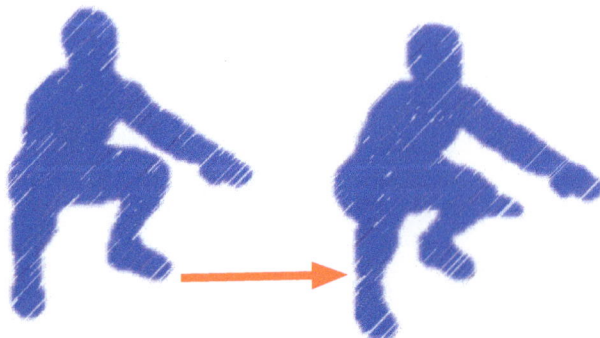

Sumo Squat

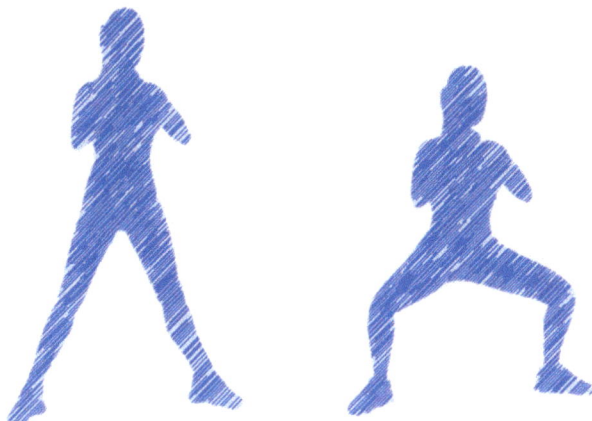

Super Skater Jump

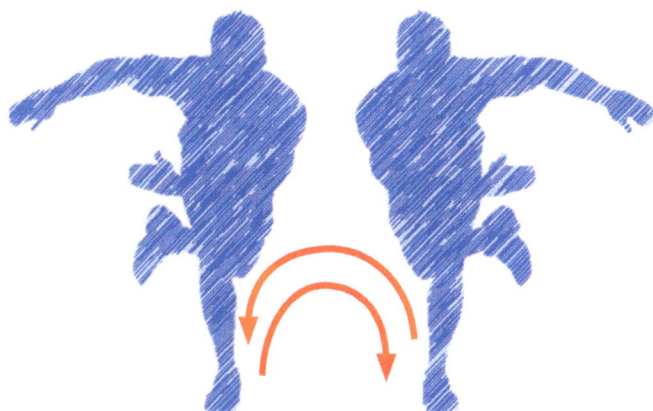

Superman

T-Rotation

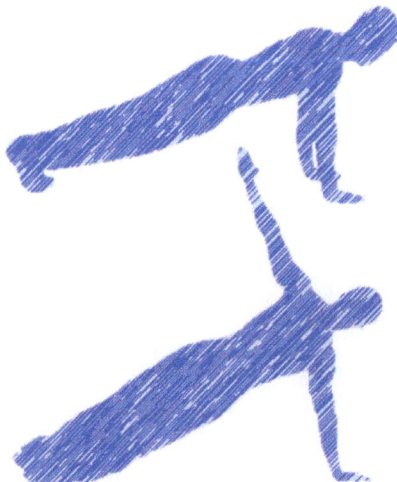

Tricep Dip

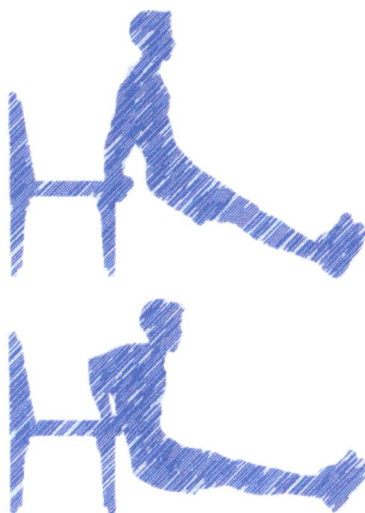

Tuck Jump

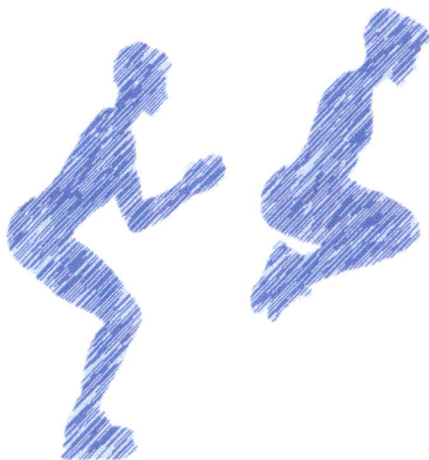

V-Up

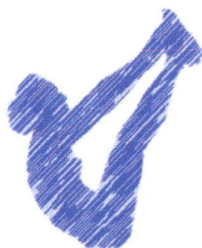

Wood Chops

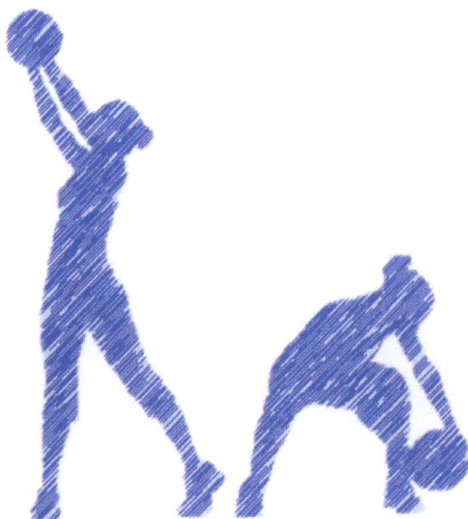

1 Leg Stand-Ups

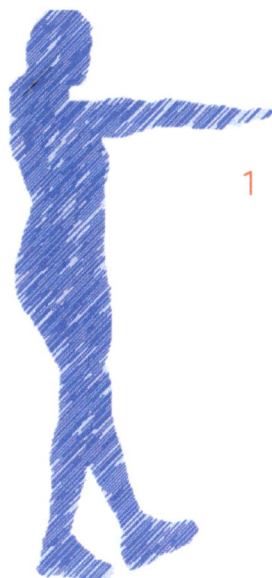

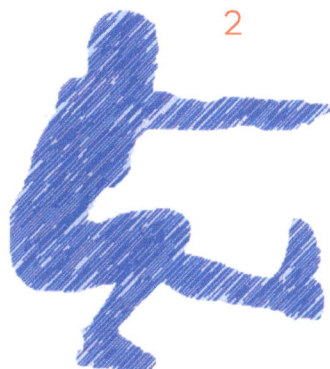

1

2